Infant Guide for New Mothers

The Best Infant Book 0-6 Months

Martha Foster

Table of Contents

Introduction

You've dived down the rabbit hole that is the internet. There is a world of information at your fingertips but it is overwhelming and, let's face it, being pregnant and getting ready to welcome a new baby into your life is already overwhelming. Opinion-based articles and product punting replaces practical information and here you are, hours into a search, still wondering what you need to do to prepare for your bundle of joy. Gone are the days of information being passed down from woman to woman, and even then, because life was so incredibly different, the village raised the baby. Grandma's advice on how to keep those cloth diapers crisp and white has been replaced with the disposable or reusable question and drinking a cup of breastfeeding brew creates question marks as to whether those products even still exist.

Being a new mom is, without any doubt, exciting but it is also a time of anxiety. Every baby is unique, no two have the same needs, but the practical information remains the same, and it is this practical information that makes new momhood a relatively pain-free transition and helps you to welcome your new life. When I set about writing this book, it was with the intention to create some structure for new moms—for them to have the village at their fingertips, cutting out the noise and external excitement of her impending new arrival. Structure, as you will quickly ascertain after bringing your baby home, is key to making it through those first glorious six months and allowing you to enjoy your baby. Now, I'm not talking about military regimented routines and hospital grade cleanliness in your home, but the kind of structure that means you will have what you need before the birth and after the homecoming will allow you to ease into motherhood and have the time to enjoy being with your bundle. Most new moms will regale you with tales of 'I wish I had known,' and it's my goal to tell you those tales, and to give you some of those answers before your baby arrives.

Transition into motherhood is not always easy and that was a lesson I learned as I journeyed through pregnancy and birth three times. I was ready, goodness knows I was ready with my first baby. I had a booming career, a stable home, had traveled and done all the things I had been told were right to do before having a child. When my first baby was born, his nursery was perfect. I had a plan for everything, right down to his birth. Little did I know that babies work on their own schedule and, six weeks before his due date, my waters broke. Frantic rushes, hospital bags not yet packed, and a birthing partner who, at 2 a.m. couldn't get his mind to kick into gear, made the frantic dash to the hospital a little chaotic. To this day, and two more babies later, I remember my mother's words of wisdom, "you won't give birth in the car. Only you may give birth in the car and that's okay, too." The irony of this wouldn't be lost on me when my second son decided to make his appearance at home only 40 minutes after my first contraction and an entire seven minutes after my waters broke. Now, as traumatic as all of that sounds, being a pragmatic planner made the chaos bearable. It meant that, although nothing went as planned, there was still a plan.

Planning ahead, knowing what your baby will need and listening to the advice of other moms is often all that will get you through the first few weeks of your baby's life. I'm not going to lie, there are days when it will all feel like it's too much, and there will be days when you wonder why you fussed at all. One thing is certain though, a little information goes a long way, and it's this critical information that I have gathered from other moms, like you, to help guide you through your first six months with your baby.

Chapter 1: Before Your Baby's Arrival

"Baby-readying your home is something that only comes much later." I've heard this so often and it is usually followed by, "I wish I had known." Not getting your home ready before your baby arrives is probably the number one mistake most expectant parents make. Waiting until your infant is moveable to baby-proof and ready your home is a common mistake, and here's why. In those first few weeks after bringing your bundle of joy home, your body will go through a couple of pretty rough phases as it adjusts to the development and birth of the baby. You're going to be sleep-deprived, possibly hormonal, and sore, no matter which type of birth you choose to have. You're going to be trying to find a routine and, hopefully, getting as much sleep as possible and, while having the perfect nursery that is social media ready is lovely, the truth is that your baby is probably going to spend more time on your chest and in your bed than in the nursery, at least for the first six weeks. Getting your home and yourself ready for your baby's arrival is going to save you time and it's going to mean that you can sleep, and bond, and allow your body to heal while you rest.

Getting Your Home Baby Ready

Choosing your baby's going home outfit, preparing photographers, and packing hospital bags are all fun but, when the time comes to welcome your baby home, certain things will need to be prepared. Regardless of what type of birth you baby choose to have, your first week to 10 days at home will need to be for you to recover and bond with your baby. Home preparation doesn't need to be stressful though and while you may not know where to start, experienced moms have weighed in on some of the tasks they completed to be home ready.

As much as I understand that you want the perfect home for your new baby, moving should be done well in advance of or only after you've had your baby and you have healed. Moving is extremely stressful and, if you feel that you absolutely must move into a new home, the second trimester is probably the best time to shift spaces. If you absolutely have to move home in the last trimester of your pregnancy, careful planning and a whole lot of hands that are not yours will need to be on deck to make your move as stress-free as possible. Regardless of whether you decide to move, investing too much time in decorating and creating a nursery is counterintuitive. The reality is that your baby will probably be sleeping in your bedroom or near you for the first few months of their lives. Decorating the nursery is more for you and less for your bundle of joy as they will only become aware of their immediate surroundings much later in their lives. If you feel the need to decorate a room to welcome your baby, rather invest in your own bedroom where you will be spending the majority of the first few months with your baby. Invest in a good breastfeeding pillow, comfortable new bedding, and practical storage solutions for those middle of the night feeds and diaper changes. Creating your own bedroom sanctuary where you feel safe, relaxed and at peace will benefit your baby as much as it does you.

While we're talking about creating a safe and relaxing space, the urge to clean will probably kick in during the last bit of your third trimester. This phenomenon, called nesting, is completely natural and will have you washing your newborn's outfits while you frantically clean cupboards and vow to not be very happy with anyone who threatens to dirty or disrupt your new nest. While there is absolutely nothing wrong with nesting, and in fact, it is incredibly useful in getting your home properly cleaned before the baby arrives, oftentimes new moms forget about the real germ magnets. Light switches, the corners of walls, door handles, the fridge door, and toilet lids often harbor germs and because we touch them regularly, may unwittingly pass these germs onto the baby and their newly developing immune system. Don't be afraid to delegate your tasks and duties to those who offer to help you. There is no need to do it all yourself. If you are concerned about harmful or harsh chemicals while cleaning, you can opt for organic, gentle products or make your own home cleaning products that are baby and mom-friendly. Don't forget to glove up while you are cleaning to prevent your hands from taking a beating.

While you are creating your bedroom sanctuary, try to declutter your space as much as possible. Storage bins and vacuum bags are a fantastic addition to every home and can be used to put away non-essentials that are not needed at the beginning of your home journey with your baby. Storing three-six months or larger clothing will mean that when you reach for an outfit, you will not need to look at sizing. If you are living in a home that has an upstairs you could delegate some storage to your downstairs area. Newborn babies can go through up to 20 diapers a day and having a downstairs or other room storage area which has diapers, rash cream, wipes, cotton wool, an additional blanket, hand cream, and nipple cream (if you are a breastfeeding mom), breast pads, spit-up cloth and spare outfits for both you and the baby could save you much needed energy. Your body will, in all likelihood, be sore postpartum and you will want to move around as little as possible. Because of this, it is sometimes easier to store these items in a box under the sofa or a table. Just make sure to purchase storage on wheels or place your storage on a rug or matt to make it easy to access. When creating your downstairs or other room storage, ensure that each bathroom is equipped with a sanitary station for yourself. This can be a storage box, basket, or bag that contains your maternity pads, disposable or maternity underwear, your sitz bath with a healing solution if you had a natural birth, breast pads, and a comfortable change of clothing in case of leaks, spills, and spit-up.

In the weeks leading up to your due date, cooking a double batch of food for storing and freezing is a great way to save time and beat the mental and physical exhaustion of having to get to the store or cook freshly made meals. Ask family and friends to bring dry goods or foods that can easily be frozen so that you have access to a wide variety of easy-to-make nutritious meals. Your body will need extra nutrition as it heals, tends to your baby, and feeds. Make sure that, if you plan on breastfeeding you can batch cook meals that are baby-friendly. Curries and chilies, while easy to make and store, can cause wind in your little one. Try to make a big batch of healing chicken soup, microwave pouches of pre-cooked oats, and rice, pre-cut and frozen fruits for breakfast oats or smoothies, and stock up on on-the-go snacks to keep your body fueled and happy. As an added extra, pre-pull cabbage leaves, spritz them with a little water, and pop them in the freezer for instant relief of sore, aching breasts when your milk comes in.

Lastly, invest in night lighting. Nasty diaper surprises, night-time clothing changes, and spit-up winding can be difficult to navigate in the middle of the night. If you are a non-breastfeeding mom, you may want to invest in a bottle and formula station that can be set up in your bedroom. Soft lighting can help to keep your baby in their sleep/wake state while you feed and helps you to navigate your room and house without waking yourself and everyone else up. If your home already comes with dimming switches, make sure that, when you settle in for the night, the switch is set to the lowest setting. Otherwise, ambient soft lighting is available in lamp form and will ensure that you can find everything you need. To make life even easier, a small bag containing everything you need to change, feed, and wind your little one can be hung or stored next to your or your baby's sleeping area.

Getting Yourself Baby Ready

Far too many moms get caught up in the baby fever of shopping and readying their home, ultimately neglecting themselves in the process. They forget that they are a marvel of nature who has grown an entire human being and that, when that little being arrives, you will nourish and care for its every need. While some of your own self-care needs have been covered in the section above, it is important that you set time aside for yourself to prepare for the changes that will happen to you.

One of the biggest concerns of a new mom is 'am I ready?' The truth is, no one will ever be completely ready for the changes that are about to happen in their life, and that's okay. Preparedness helps to ease into the transition a little more seamlessly and can help new moms to enjoy those first few weeks with their baby without having to worry about the small things. Some of this advice is practical, while some will support you emotionally, both of which are important in their own way.

Before your due date, some practical items will be needed for yourself. Gift giving and baby registries are great but don't forget to add your own self-care items to those lists. Try to have your baby shower towards the beginning of your third trimester so that there is still time to get to the store for the additional items you need before the weight and busyness of the last few weeks kicks in. Dedicate a shelf or drawer for a new refreshed 'fourth-trimester' wardrobe. This can include comfortable, loose-fitting clothing that will keep you relaxed but will also help you while your body transitions back to its post-baby shape. Tights, leggings, loose-fitting nursing shirts or t-shirts, loose-fitting dresses with adjustable or loosening straps, and nursing bras that are a size or two larger than the bra you are currently wearing are all great additions to your new mom wardrobe. If your baby is a winter baby, slip ons, nice thick socks, and a warm oversized nightgown that your baby can be slipped into are an essential for night-time feeds.

Try to purchase as many disposable or inexpensive comfortable washable panties as possible. The normal period for postpartum bleeding is four weeks but can last for up to 12 weeks. Sanitary pads should be bought in varying sizes and thicknesses. While the majority of the large, ultra-absorbent pads will be used in the first 10 days, sometimes your lochia blood flow, can return and become heavier for a day or two, especially as your milk comes in or your baby increases their feeds. The majority of your sanitary wear will be midflow but it's wise to also invest in a two-week supply of panty liners for the last few weeks of your postpartum bleeding. Don't worry about having too many sanitary pads. You will not be using tampons or internal menstruation protection for your postpartum or the first cycle after your baby is born, and panty liners make great backup breast pads to prevent leaks. Cesarean moms often opt to use mid-sized or thick sanitary pads to protect and offer a soft layer between their incision and their underwear to ease discomfort. Most hospitals will provide cesarean section moms with a pair of compression stockings but having one or two spare pairs is great for when your current pair is in the washer. It is important for natural birth moms to also purchase a pair of compression stockings as birth can be unpredictable and a person can never be assured that things will go to plan.

Both c section and natural birth moms will need some level of at-home wound care. This will differ, depending on the type of birth you have elected to have, but as we said before, it is never a bad idea for you to plan for both types of births. Antiseptic cream helps to keep c section wounds clean and sterile and some brands come with anesthetic properties. You can always consult your gynecologist before the birth of your baby as to which over-the-counter product they prefer. For natural birth moms, there are a host of new hygiene products on the market that promote vaginal healing. A sitz bath or small tub can be used to splash sterile hygiene solutions or a weak salt water solution onto the perineum and vulva. Do not use any product that pushes water or solutions into the vagina as this can introduce bacteria into your uterus while it heals. Wound care doesn't start and end with the body part from which your baby emerged. Investing in relaxing shower washes and lotions are a wonderful way to feel refreshed and attractive again as your body readjusts. You will not be allowed to have a bath, or soak in a tub for some time so avoid soaking products and opt for soothing evening shower gels or refreshing morning scents to invigorate yourself. Most moms will suffer from dry skin and excessive hair loss in the first few weeks postpartum. This is completely normal and can be managed with moisturizing balms and deep conditioning treatments. When purchasing your self-care products, don't forget to add breast and nipple relief products to your list. Pre-frozen cabbage is an age-old, tried and tested method of soothing hot, aching breasts, while lanolin can be used on cracked or sore nipples to relieve pain.

Your nutrition needs to be maintained and, for breastfeeding moms, calorie intake will need to be upped slightly to accommodate feeding your baby. Stocking up on nutritious snacks is one way to keep your body healthy and energized but pregnancy supplementation should not be stopped altogether. If you no longer wish to take prenatal vitamins, you can shop around for vitamins that are specifically designed for the postnatal period. Postnatal vitamins may include more iron but most post- and prenatal vitamins have the same ingredients. If you opt for an iron-rich supplement, don't forget to up your fiber intake or ensure that you have a natural bowel relief product on hand to counteract constipation. If you choose to breastfeed your baby, ensure that your supplementation list includes raspberry leaf tea and fennel to help your milk supply along.

The first few weeks after bringing your baby home often passes in a blur of feeding, bathing, changing, and visitors. Seasoned moms will tell you that, beyond the practical clothing, wound care, and self-care items, boundaries are going to be your number one sanity saver. Oftentimes, new moms are not sure how to express their wishes prior to their baby being born, and a constant stream of visitors and well-wishers can become overwhelming, interrupting routines, cutting into your much-needed sleep time and, no matter how well-intentioned they may be, will cause more stress than is needed. When my second son was born, I had set all the healthy boundaries I thought I needed to make sure that the first six weeks with him were about bonding and finding a routine that worked for him and my eldest son. What I hadn't counted on was that, while my first child was born in the middle of summer, my second was born in winter, when it was raining and muddy. Suddenly, glasses of cold water which could just be rinsed and put in the dishwasher were replaced with mugs that held coffee, and side plates that piled up with the remnants of welcome baby cake. My house was constantly muddy with trails of dried grit through to my bedroom where my bundle of joy slept. It felt like I spent endless amounts of time getting rid of grit, hardened mud, and packing the dishwasher. When my last baby was born, I made sure to set additional boundaries to preserve my sleep time. I purchased disposable plates for snacks. Whenever possible, I asked that guests bring a pizza so that the leftovers could be frozen for my older kids. I asked that shoes be left at the door to prevent mud from being traipsed through our home and that mugs or cups be rinsed and washed. Sticking to a specific set of visiting times is a great idea. It helps to stem the flow of people through your house. This allows you to maintain a routine with your baby, and means you can move your baby to a visiting room to reduce the introduction of dirt into your sleeping area. Think about who was a calming influence on you before giving birth and ask them if they would like to be your dedicated caregiver during specific times of the week so that you can have a shower that is more than two minutes long or a decent amount of uninterrupted sleep. Assigning some money to that person to pick up milk, bread, or other consumables that run out or spoil will also negate delivery people at your door while you are in the middle of a feed or sleeping. While these may all seem like trivial things, the time you save adds up and allows you more time during the first few days to take care of yourself as well.

Lastly, take time to prepare for the birth of the baby. Create a birthing plan and then create a contingency plan. Make sure this is packed in your hospital bag and ensure that your birthing partner knows and can be your advocate for both your best and worst-case birthing scenarios. Remember to include your birthing partner's wishes in your plan and what you would like to happen with your baby following the birth. If you find yourself overwhelmed, create a list of questions and, in a quiet moment, answer those questions to formulate your birthing plan. How do I want to labor? Where should my birthing partner be? Do I want music or meditation guiding? Who will cut my baby's cord? Do I want my baby placed directly on my chest with the cord still attached? Who will be with my baby should they need to be taken to NICU? Who is my second choice doctor? These are all questions that can help you formulate a good set of birthing plans which will make the moment of birth easier to handle. Don't forget to include your immediate postnatal period in hospital or at home, and if you have elected for a home birth, needs. When you are shopping for yourself and your baby, take your birth plan along and include an item to spoil yourself for bringing a beautiful new life into this world and being an incredible, strong human being.

Chapter 2: Shopping for Your Baby

New moms often fall into the trap of owning entirely too many outfits; we have, after all, imagined welcoming our new bundle of joy into our lives for almost a full nine months. While cute outfits and nursery bedding are nice to have, the reality is that you will probably have more outfits than your growing infant can wear once your baby shower has come and gone. I've seen it happen almost every time a mom hits the store, the aisles of color-coded tops and bottoms lure moms in. Trust me when I say that being pragmatic when you're doing your own shopping is the way to go. That's not to say that you shouldn't splurge on the things you really want but oftentimes creating a practical wardrobe and baby essentials rack is far more important. By week four, you'll be rewashing those favorite onesies while frilly dresses, bow ties, and britches will be boxed for memories.

Baby Essentials

Every seasoned mom wishes that they had a checklist that told them exactly what to buy for their baby. Now, I'm not talking about those generalized lists that tell you how many of each item to purchase but rather a comprehensive guide as to what will be needed daily for each stage of your baby's life. These items should be bought to make your life easier, and while we understand that picking a going home item is important, at some point the novelty of your baby looking social media ready is replaced with, 'looks great AND is practical.' A lot of what we cover in this chapter will be based on your personal preferences but each section is broken down to allow you the choice to purchase those items.

Daytime Clothing

Daytime is when you can dress your baby up into those cute outfits you received at your baby shower or that you just couldn't resist adding to your baby's closet. Cute outfits like baby jeans and separate jackets are adorable when on but can be impractical for diaper changes in the middle of the night. Your baby's clothing will depend on the season and whether or not they are a warm or a cold baby. In the beginning, your baby will be dressed in layers until you have been able to ascertain how well they maintain their body temperature. The general rule is that your baby should be dressed in one layer more than you, but again, this will be largely dependent on how well your baby maintains their temperature and whether they generally run warm or cold. Winter babies should never leave the home without a bonnet or hat and socks and the quantities in this list should be doubled for these items. Short-sleeved vests can be replaced with long-sleeved vests depending on the season and your own requirements. Your little one will probably be in onesies until the cord has fully detached from them and pants or separate outfits should be avoided to prevent irritation to the umbilical area for the first week to 10 days. Try to be prepared with three tiny baby or premature baby outfits as often birth weights are incorrect and your baby may be lighter than expected.

Table 1. Daytime Clothing Checklist

8 x Vests	5 x Onesies
5 x Pants (After the cord has detached)	5 x Cardigans or jackets (Double for winter baby)

4 x Dress up outfits (This is optional)	3 x Hats or bonnets (Double for winter baby)
8 x Socks	3 x Hand mittens (Double for winter baby)
2 x Snowsuits or weather suits for winter baby	2 x Wide brimmed sun hats for a summer baby
Infant laundry detergent and softener	

Nighttime Clothing

Nighttime clothing for your baby needs to be practical to allow for quick diaper and clothing changes. This keeps your baby in a sleepy state and ensures that, once your feed is complete, you can get some much-needed sleep. Not knowing if your baby is too hot or too cold at night is probably one of the biggest concerns new moms face and it often leads to sleepless nights as moms fuss and check over their sleeping baby. The general rule of thumb of one layer more than you is useful for night dressing but your blankets and home heating should be taken into account as well. For temperatures of 75 degrees Fahrenheit or higher, babies should be in one layer of light clothing and a light swaddle or cotton sleeping bag. For temperatures from 70 to 75 degrees Fahrenheit, one layer of light clothing and a pair of long pants or a light full-sleeved onesie with a light swaddle or cotton sleeping bag. For standard temperatures of 59 to 70 degrees Fahrenheit, you should have two layers of clothing, a short-sleeved vest for higher temperatures and a long sleeve vest for lower temperatures and one additional layer of long-sleeved / pants clothing, and a lightly padded sleeping bag or mid-thickness swaddle. For temperatures of below 59 degrees Fahrenheit, your baby should remain in layers of long-sleeved clothing but the sleeping bag or swaddle should be thick to retain heat. Sleeping bags or sacks are great for three to six-month-old babies who have discovered their feet and begin to fight their swaddle or wriggle out of their blanket. If your baby is a particularly restless sleeper who slips into their sleeping bag, thermal onesies can be worn as an additional layer, or nightgowns can be used to easily change night time diapers.

Table 1. Night Time Clothing List

8 vests short or long-sleeved depending on the season	8 onesies - the zippered ones are a lifesaver
4 tops long sleeve as an additional layer (optional)	4 bottoms longs as an additional layer (optional)
4 baby stretch nightgowns (optional)	5 swaddles - thickness depending on the season
2 sleeping sacks or bags - thickness depending on the season	

Feeding

Other than sleeping, your little one will spend most of their time feeding. Breastfeeding moms can often feel like they are stuck in an endless cycle of feeding and changing, and fitting in other household chores or time for themselves can be challenging. This is because nursing, breastfed babies often take longer to get their fill, especially when they are going through a growth spurt. We will cover more on feeding later, but finding a feeding routine that works for you, regardless of whether or not your baby breast or bottle feeds, can be made easier. An enormous amount of money does not need to be spent initially on your baby's feeding equipment. Remember, we told you every baby is different and bottle-fed babies may take time to choose which bottle, nipple, or formula they prefer. Likewise, with breastfed babies who are being fed with nipple shields, some experimentation may be needed to find what works best for both mom and baby. As with your birth, prepare for both types of feeds. One never knows what will work for your tiny tyke or yourself until you have begun feeding. Your single largest investment in feeding your baby will be a breast pump. Almost every area has breast pump rental equipment which you can try out before taking the leap and investing in a pump of your own. For moms who opt to bottle feed, a hand-held pump is still a rentable necessity so that you can pump a small amount of milk to prevent engorgement, milk fever, and extremely sore, full breasts. Breastfeeding tops are great for both bottle and breast moms as they add an extra layer of protection to your baby when they are strapped to you while you are out and about, or to soothe overstimulated babies who need to be removed from light and noise while not at home. Please keep in mind that breastfed babies usually get all of the vitamins and minerals they need from healthy moms with the exception of vitamin D. This is especially true for babies born in winter or in the Northern Hemisphere and, because of this, the AAP, (American Academy of Paediatrics) recommends that breastfed babies receive vitamin D supplements for the first year of their life or until vitamin D can be introduced into their diet after six months of age.

Table 3. Feeding Essentials

Breastpump, rent until you find one that works	2 Bottles - choose 4 teats/nipples that can be interchanged
Breastmilk freezer bags or storage	1 Box of two different types of formula
2 Nipple shields - short term solution	2 Large boxes of breast pads
Microwave sterilizer or baby-safe solution, bottle brush, and teat brush	Lanolin cream for sore nipples
2 Breastfeeding shirts to place over clothing	4 Nursing bras
8 Spit Up cloths	Pediatric vitamin D drops & gripe water

Diaper Changing

Breastfed babies will have more soiled diapers daily than formula-fed babies. This is because breastmilk is more easily digested than formula and, as such, moves through the baby's system quicker. On average, you can expect to use 12 diapers per day in the newborn phase for a breastfed baby and eight diapers a day for a formula-fed baby. Whether you use reusable diapers or disposable diapers is entirely up to you but, should you decide to use reusable diapers, a small pack of disposables is suggested for trips out of your home. Diaper sizing generally goes up by weight category and often, newborn diapers are only needed for the first two weeks. In general, you will use more size 2 (12 to 18 pounds) and size 4 (22 to 37 pounds) diapers in the first six months of your baby's life than any other size. Most stores will return and swap out unopened packs of disposable diapers, so don't worry about having too many diapers for your little one.

Table 4. Diaper Changing Needs

30 Reusable diapers	15 Waterproof diaper covers for reusable diapers
5 Large packs of diaper liners	5 Diaper snappies or safety pins for reusable diapers
1 Big box of baking soda to neutralize the acid in reusable diapers when washing	3 Packs of newborn disposable diapers or 1 pack for reusable moms

1 Pack disposable changing pads or 2 washable changing pads	2 Tubs of diaper barrier cream
5 Packs of disposable wipes (sensitive) or 12 diaper reusable washcloths	

Bathing

Bathing my babies was always a special time of bonding even if it was slightly trickier in winter to get the ambient temperature right. When my first baby was born, I had every baby cologne, baby lotion, and potion available on the market to make sure my little one smelled amazing. This backfired hugely when I realized his sensitive skin did not tolerate anything that was heavily perfumed and, ultimately, when my other kids were born, I dumped the idea of sweet-smelling babies and opted for practical, neutral products designed for babies with sensitive skin. One thing I didn't realize the first time around is that babies don't need a lot of products and eventually, to prevent the products from spoiling, I ended up using them on myself. Try, wherever possible, to exclude baby products from your shower registry and buy them yourself so that you can be sure of the ingredients. Most brands now offer 'top-to-toe' options for bathing which saves space and time when bathing your little one. How often to bathe your baby is entirely up to you and I found it was very much season-dependent. My summer newborn required daily bathing whereas my winter babies only needed to be bathed three times a week. You will find what works for you and your baby, depending on how hot or cold the temperature is, how often they spit up, and how sensitive their skin is to cleansing lotions.

Table 5. Bathing

5 Reusable washcloths or 5 packs of cotton wool pads	2 Bottles of top-to-toe wash
1 Bottle of baby shampoo and 1 bottle of baby wash (If not using top-to-toe)	1 Large tub of unscented aqueous cream
1 Bottle baby powder (for summer babies to prevent chubby chafe)	1 Small pack of Q-tips for umbilical care
1 Small bottle of surgical spirits for umbilical care	3 Hooded baby towels
1 Baby hairbrush (keeps cradle cap at bay)	1 Approved baby bath support device

Sleeping and Soothing

Every baby soothes differently. Some prefer to be swaddled, while others will refuse to have their arms and legs gently wrapped. As a mom, you will learn what works best for you and your baby. Most new moms spend an exorbitant amount of time and effort into a nursery which will probably not be used for the first six months other than for storage. Your greatest investment for your baby's sleeping needs will be a good quality crib and mattress. When selecting a crib, think about the years to come and opt for one which can be easily converted into a toddler bed as your baby grows. The spacing between the crib bars should be narrow. While crib bumpers and duvets are pretty, they are impractical and are ultimately a waste of money as your baby will not need them and many of the products out there are a danger to your baby from a suffocation point of view. If you are a breastfeeding mom, you may find that co-sleeping works better for you. Co-sleeping products can range from 'in-bed' sleep nests to Moses baskets and open-sided cribs which can be attached to your bed. Deciding which one works best for you and your baby will require a little research so don't forget to reach out to experienced co-sleeping moms for their tips, tricks, and recommendations.

Table 6. Sleeping Essentials

Good quality crib (preferably extendable to a toddler bed)	A good breathable quality mattress
3 Approved breathable waterproof mattress savers or 1 pack of disposable changing pads	3 Breathable fitted sheets for your mattress
3 Large cotton blankets	8 Swaddles or receiving blankets

Approved breastfeeding pillows for co-sleeping breastfeeding moms	2 Pacifiers of a different brand until your baby chooses their favorite

Healthcare

Nobody likes to think that their baby may become sick but the reality is that, sometimes, you will need a little extra help to soothe your baby, especially with winter colds coming into play and teething, which can occur any time from three months onwards. Not all healthcare needs for your baby will mean that they are sick, but having some general supplies on hand is never a bad idea.

Table 7. Medical Needs

Pediatric rectal or ear thermometer	Bulb syringe for suctioning mucus
Pediatric medicine dropper or an eyedropper	Pediatric fever medication
Pediatric constipation suppositories	Nail clippers or baby emery board

Probably the most neglected and most hotly contested essentials you will need for every day and on the go will be these essentials. Some moms will swear that a good quality reclinable stroller is essential from day one while others swear that a good quality baby wrap is what is needed. For me, I preferred to have my babies strapped to me. This allowed me to carry on with everyday tasks, knowing that my baby was close and protected. Some of these items are absolute must-haves while others will be purely based on preference but all will be well used by the time your baby is six months old. Some of these essentials, like your baby's car seat-carrier have to be purchased before the baby's arrival as hospitals, rightfully, do not allow any baby to be discharged without a proper vehicle carrier.

Table 8. Everyday Items

Approved infant car seat	Sun visor for car
Reclinable stroller	Baby wrap
Baby monitor	Portable heater to warm the bathroom for bathing time
Night lighting	Room thermometer
Thermal bottle warmer	Freezable Teethers

Diaper bag or backpack	

What Should or Could be Avoided

The amount of merchandise available to new moms is, as we have established, overwhelming. While shopping for my last baby I was struck by just how many ridiculously overpriced and utterly useless some of these goods were. Getting lost in a maze of diaper rash applicators, diaper changing gloves and automatic formula makers had me wondering how on earth these items are ever sold. The reality check came when I realized that some of these products—I'm looking at you shopping cart covers—had trapped me as a first-time mom. The reality is, baby products and furniture are a money-making scheme, and many of the things that are "nice to have" end up collecting dust in the corner of a room or lost in the back of a cupboard, its days numbered by plans for your next garage sale. Other items are incredibly nice to have and will ultimately serve their purpose long after your baby is born and, because of this, one should look at longevity. These longer use items include your baby's nursery and crib; rocking chairs can be replaced with comfortable recliners which, if a quality piece of furniture is bought, could still be in use when your baby becomes a teenager in the years to come. When diving into the maze of nice-to-haves ask yourself the question of whether this will be an immediate need, a need within a few months, few years, or will I ever use this at all.

Things like play mobiles and walking rings are nice to have but will only be needed in a few months as your baby will neither be mobile nor aware of their surroundings for quite some time. In the same way, playpens and baby gates are absolutely not a necessity until your baby shows signs of wanting to move around. Other items, such as a portable baby bath, seem to have become a staple to many new moms but by the 3rd or 4th bath, you will realize how cumbersome and ungainly they are and will instead plop the baby in the main tub in their baby support device. This is not to say that portable baths are not useful, especially for homes and apartments which only have a shower but a much smaller, round tub works just as well, holds less water, and is easier to drain. Likewise, a reclinable stroller may not be a necessity for some moms but, for myself, I bought a good quality stroller and had breathable foam made to create a padded inner so that my baby could sleep next to my side of the bed for the first six weeks. It made feeding easier and negated that need for a Moses basket or bassinet. You will need to 'feel out' which of the nice to haves fit-your-lifestyle and which are headed for the 'I shouldn't have bought that pile'.

Table 9. Nice to Have

Portable baby bath	Diaper changing table (any set of drawers with a changing matt will do)
Rocking chair or recliner	Playpen (can be bought later)
Baby gates (can be bought later)	Baby walker (can be bought later)
Baby rattles (can be bought later)	Mobiles

Baby rocker/glider (never leave your baby unattended in a rocker/glider)	A reclining stroller (lifestyle dependent)

Table 10. Absolutely No Need

Plastic baby clothes hangers	Shoes
White noise machine (the internet has plenty of free options)	Disposable wipe warmer or dirty diaper gloves
Pacifier case (resealable plastic bags and breastmilk bags do the same thing)	Pacifier wipes
Bathtub thermometer	Shopping cart seat covers (wear your baby instead, it's safer)
Diaper cream dispenser	Diaper Bin
Formula mixer	Crib bedding sets

Chapter 3: Hello Baby - The Basics

You have prepared and the day has finally arrived to meet your baby. Initially, at birth, you may have feelings of being completely overwhelmed or even detached. This is all completely normal as your body deals with the rush of hormones and natural chemicals that help a woman to heal and provide nourishment for their baby after birth. Perhaps you are feeling a sense of disappointment that your birth didn't go as planned and that is understandable. Over the next few days, you will spend your time recovering and getting to know your baby. For the most part, a new mom will feel an instant connection to their baby but, for some moms, this connection can only come later. There is absolutely nothing wrong with not connecting with your little one immediately but if these feelings of disconnection are accompanied by sadness, of being excessively overwhelmed, or of harming yourself or your baby, you should consult your gynecologist immediately, as you may be suffering from postpartum depression, a fairly common disorder that can affect even the most seasoned mothers. Far too many moms feel enormous pressure to get on with their lives. Streams of visitors, the need to have a perfectly clean house, and store visits can all add extra pressure to an already stressful situation. During your first six weeks with your baby, you will spend most of your time getting to know the tiny person you have brought into the world. Every baby is unique, and so your approach to your baby will need to be unique to everyone else's. Your little angel and you will have to learn to fall into your own routine that suits both of your needs. While the uniqueness of you and your baby can never be overlooked, experienced moms will tell you that there are some essentials that you need to know that will help you transition into motherhood.

Getting to Know Your Baby

Babies are marvels of nature. They are delicate but not fragile. They instinctively know what is needed to survive and demand those things without question. Your first few hours and days will probably be spent taking in your baby's features, trying to ascertain who they look like more. As time passes, you will begin to notice the smaller details and, for some moms, these details can be alarming. If something is really bothering you, please consult your physician, pediatrician, or midwife, but for the most part, all newborn babies are temporarily marred by bruises, birthmarks and other apparent minor deformities.

I remember my first newborn son being brought to me after our initial bonding time, changing him and gasping in horror at the mark on his arm. Frantically, I called the nurse to ask what they had done to my baby. She lovingly explained that some vaccinations cause hotspots and the mark on his arm were as a result of his vitamin K injection and his required vaccination. I wasn't impressed but accepted that it was required. Later, when the pediatrician visited and performed my baby's physical examination, I was less impressed. This examination is, of course, necessary, but as a first-time mom, I felt an overwhelming need to smack the doctor's hands away to protect my newborn. Ultimately, the physical, which checks your newborn's hips, joints, eyes, ears, heart, and for little boys, testicles, does your baby no harm and I learned, with my subsequent babies, to remove myself from the room when this physical exam was performed. When it came time for the first bath, I was adamant that I would be present. Now I had seen umbilical cords before but they were generally a few days old and well on their way to drying out. Nothing prepared me for the strange blue, grey hue of the plump cord coming from my baby's navel. How the nurse gently flopped the plastic clipped from side to side to clean the area where it joined my son's belly made me queasy. I wondered if I would ever be able to get used to having to keep his cord clean and dry for it to heal. By the time it did eventually fall off, I was a pro, and the fact that I was so incredibly aware of whether it was making my baby uncomfortable made me a little fastidious about making sure it was clean, dry, and irritant-free at all times. The point is, don't be horrified if you feel queasy or uneasy about cleaning your baby's cord. Keeping it clean, dry and diaper irritation-free will mean that it will fall between seven and 10 days after your baby's birth and your little one will be sporting a new belly button. Should there be any redness, bleeding, or discharge from your baby's cord as it is healing, please contact your healthcare provider to make sure there isn't an infection.

Speaking of the first seven days, your baby will undergo some strange transformations. Some babies may be born with breasts, and little girls may have some bloody vaginal discharge. This is a result of your hormones and is nothing to be alarmed about. As your little one begins to adjust to life outside of the womb, their own hormones will kick in and their body will correct any hormonal imbalances. Your perfect newborn's skin may begin to dry, peel, or slough off as they develop the protective barrier that is needed to keep their skin from being damaged easily. This sloughing phase can last longer with premature babies whose skin is very thin, sensitive, and easily damaged. It is extremely important to stay away from heavily scented products or products that are not specifically designed for baby use so that you do not irritate their skin. Some babies may be born with long fingernails that will peel off between Day 5 and Day 10. Again, this is nothing to be alarmed about and is usually just an indication that your baby was slightly overdue. There may be some swelling and bruising on your baby's body and head, their head may be oddly cone-shaped, or your baby's eyes may be bloodshot for the first 10 days post-birth as well. This is very common for babies who have been born naturally because of the pressure caused by squeezing and pushing during birth. If your baby needed to be assisted at birth with the use of forceps or a ventouse, they will be more likely to have marks on their head, face, or body. C-section babies may also have these marks due to the external force required to get them out through such a small incision. Once again, if you are particularly worried about a mark you see on your baby or are unhappy with how they are moving their limbs, speak to your midwife or pediatrician. Most birth bruises and marks will disappear after 10 days and you will be able to see whether your little one has been endowed with any other birthmarks. Most commonly, newborns will present with a red or pink 'V' on their forehead, but this can sometimes be present on the upper eyelid and neck. These were once called 'stork marks', a homage to the old wives' tale that the stork brought babies to their mother. You may notice small raised dark or bright red areas on your baby's face or body. These are called infantile haemangioma, although I prefer the less scary common name, 'strawberries'. Again, this is completely normal and, while they may grow slightly larger as your baby grows, they will eventually fade away entirely. Be aware that strawberries are usually present from birth and are very localized to their area. If your newborn develops a rash or becomes fussy and isn't feeling well, consult your physician immediately.

Ask any mother what their biggest fears were with their newborn and three common concerns come up but the resounding fear winner has to be, 'soft spots.' Called fontanelles, these are the two dents on the top and the back of your baby's head where the skull has not yet fused together. These non-fused skull bones are there to assist your baby in squeezing through the birth canal and to facilitate the rapid growth of your baby's brain. Many moms are terrified that they will cause damage to their newborn by pressing too hard on the fontanelle, and while it is true that some damage can be caused by extreme or excessive pressure, the soft spots are protected with a tough membrane to prevent damage to your baby's brain. Washing your baby's hair or bruising with a baby brush will not cause harm to your baby. Another fear of new moms is their baby's eyes. For the first two or so weeks of your baby's life, their vision will be unfocused and will need time to develop and become used to the outside world. At around two weeks, you may notice your baby's eyes doing strange things as they begin to focus on you or surrounding sounds. Squinting, eye-rolling and fluttering are all normal newborn eye reflexes that will begin to normalize at around three months. To help your baby focus, try holding objects or your face approximately 8 inches, (20cm) from their face. This is within their vision distance path and will prevent them from having to strain. If your baby's eyes do not return to their normal position, or if eye reflexes have not slowed considerably by three months, consult your pediatrician. Vision and focus may take longer in premature babies though and age adjustment should be considered. Last on the list of common concerns is your newborn's reflexes. Remember when I told you that your baby is a marvelous creation? Newborn's come with a set of reflexes that help them survive. Common reflexes, such as moving towards whatever has brushed their cheek or opening their mouth with a cheek or lip brush, are your baby's way of telling you they are hungry. This natural reflex triggers them to suck. During the first few days of your baby's life, they will learn how to coordinate breathing and sucking together, so if your baby double breathes, or seems to skip a breath while feeding it is only because they are still learning to do both things at once. Finger grasping, and startle reflexes, which happen when your baby suddenly jerks and moves to grab you, are also normal and will begin to disappear as your baby gets older. Most of these initial survival reflexes, except sucking, will disappear over the first few months of your baby's life and will be replaced with the conscious thought patterns that you will teach your little one.

The Essentials and When to Call Your Doctor

Many of the essentials touched on in the section will be discussed in-depth in future chapters, but for now, let's talk about your baby. Babies cry a lot, eat even more, and sleep an incredible amount of the time in their first six weeks. This is because their little body has quite a bit of growing to get done in those first few weeks after birth and by six months old, your little one would have grown between half and a full inch and gained between 5 and 7 ounces each and every month. This means that their little body needs a whole lot of fuel to accommodate their physical and mental growth. There will be times where you put your baby down to nap and when they wake, you will be convinced their face has changed or that they feel heavier, and you would probably be right. Because your little angel is a growing machine, you will need to make sure that you try and institute routines right as soon as you can. Breastfed babies will need to drink every two to three hours, and that means setting your alarm clock at night, Momma, because believe it or not, some babies sleep through from Day 1. This is not ideal however because of the risk of blood sugar dips. Many breastfeeding moms choose to feed 'on-demand' and that is fine if it works for you. The biggest complaint I hear from moms who breastfeed is that it is a commitment and that, quite often, they feel like all they are doing during the day is feeding their baby. If you choose to 'baby-lead' breastfeed your baby, you can try wearing your baby at other times of the day so that you can get some things done during your baby's nap times. Formula-fed babies require feeds every three to four hours, depending on the instructions on the formula tin or box. It is of utmost importance that you do not deviate from these instructions as formula is specifically designed to be mixed with distilled or parboiled water in those ratios to ensure your baby gets all of the vitamins they need.

By the time your baby gets to four weeks you will have ascertained what your routine is and, barring the occasional growth spurt, will be able to begin getting your life back, setting aside your own nap, shower, and chore times. By week 4, your body will also be feeling stronger and your hormones would have settled to a certain extent. The important thing to remember during this four and eight-week period is that there may be days between where your baby is more alert and awake, and their appetite will mean they will demand more frequent and longer feeds. This is just their body getting ready for a growth spurt and, with a little patience, you will both settle back into your routine once they have received the fuel they need. During your first few weeks, try to embrace the chaos that comes with having a baby. Understand that nothing bad will happen if you don't bathe them daily and the majority of people will understand if your hair is about four days overdue a wash. It takes a couple of weeks, and sometimes a couple of tries to institute a routine that works for both of you. The important thing is that you and your baby get a good amount of rest and an even better amount of time to get to know each other as this will allow you to know if there is something that needs changing or if there is something wrong with your baby.

Should you ever be unsure of whether you or your baby need medical care, do not brush it off. If your bleeding increases, if you pass clots larger than a grape, or if you feel light-headed, have a persistent headache, or are seeing stars or an aura, contact your health physician immediately. Postpartum birth complications, while rare, can happen and should not be taken lightly. Likewise, a little weepiness and feeling sad is normal after having a baby but, sometimes, those feelings are amplified and may require a visit to your physician. Postpartum depression is a very real syndrome and should not be taken lightly. A baby who is fussy, feverish, develops a rash, is congested, or has too many lapses in breathing should be seen by a pediatrician immediately. Green stool that is runny, or is filled with mucus, grey or white stool should also not be taken lightly. Babies dehydrate incredibly quickly and diarrhea is the number one cause of dehydration in infants. Finally, while it is completely normal for a baby to turn a little yellow and be slightly jaundiced after birth, persistent jaundice, yellowing of the eyes, and light, grey, or white stool is a sign of acute yellow jaundice and the baby should be seen by a physician immediately. Including vitamin D in your baby's daily milk intake and light sunning through a closed window is a good way to reverse or prevent minor jaundice in infants.

Recovering From a Difficult Birth

I found out I was pregnant with my last baby just shy of my 40th birthday. I was terrified. Growing up in a society that deems pregnant mothers as 'geriatric' once they reach the age of 35, being in a foreign country where English is barely spoken, and knowing there was a big possibility my husband would need to return to work before our baby was born threw me into a tizz. Once the dust had settled though, I reminded myself that I was a veteran at this. I had given birth without my husband before and had managed a newborn and another child with the experience I had gained. And then the global pandemic hit. The chance to give birth in a country that did have English as a first language became impossible but at least my husband was homebound and that meant he would, at least, get to experience the birth of one of our children. Throughout my pregnancy, I readied myself, making plans for who would look after our other children, planning hospital routes, and memorizing numbers of how to get to the hospital in the midst of lockdowns and curfews. I began nesting, setting boundaries, and ordering online, knowing that organizing for this new edition would take a little more planning and forethought. What was a relatively easy pregnancy took a strange turn around 32 weeks when I became ill. Hanging over the toilet after every meal became the norm and because of the delicate healthcare situation with the pandemic, I was not permitted to see a doctor unless it was an emergency or I was in labor. When I eventually did see the doctor, five weeks later, my life was turned upside down. The hour following my appointment was IV drips, medications, and worried expressions. My blood pressure was so high that the doctors feared I would have a stroke. I messaged my husband, telling him to get to the hospital and to bring the hospital bag as I was sure our son would be born that day. In the middle of the phone call, alarms went off and I was whisked off to surgery. I shouted. Screamed for anyone to listen to me or to understand what I was saying. I wanted a natural birth. Why were they taking me in for a c-section? While a stern old man stuck a needle into my spine, the surgeon arrived to tell me our son's heart had stopped and that although it was now beating, his heartbeat was way too low and he wouldn't survive if they didn't get

42

him out immediately. And so, 1 hour and 45 minutes after my routine final trimester check-up, our 3-pound IUGR son was born. I lay numbly on the table, violated, weeping, wondering what I could have done to keep him in longer. His father had missed his birth. My body felt like it wasn't mine as it was being sewn together and, unlike my other two births, a brand new screaming baby was not placed on my chest but rather whisked away to the NICU. I would spend a further four days in ICU battling high blood pressure, sobbing to see my child or my husband. I was isolated from the world. Isolated from my family and no one spoke my language. The messages from well-wishers read that they were glad we were both alive but the fact remained that I had not seen my son. By Day 6, my husband was permitted into the hospital to fetch me and it was only then that we were allowed to see our baby. He went on to spend a further seven weeks in NICU before coming home. In that time my milk came in and as much as I expressed, it dried up. I missed our baby's first smile, his first bath, and even his first dreaded bowel movement. I was bitter, angry, and thoroughly heartbroken. Nothing had gone to plan. My baby wasn't home. My children were disappointed they couldn't meet their brother and I was only permitted one hour per day to visit my newborn because of the pandemic. I couldn't smell his tiny head, or place him on my breast. Finally, our baby came home, some two months later and I began to heal as I soaked him and got into the routines of a newborn.

Birth is a difficult process to heal from even if things go exactly as you have planned. Your body will be sore. You will be more tired and fatigued than you have ever been in your life and, when you add hormones and baby blues into the mix, the first four weeks after your baby is born has the potential to turn into a highly volatile situation. When your birth did not go as planned, it is normal to feel a sense of loss. You will grieve the ideas you had for your perfect birth and for your ideal homecoming. Overcoming difficult childbirth is all too often downplayed as baby blues but it is an enormous loss. One that deserves your time and attention to overcome. You may carry around feelings of resentment, failure, or guilt and these feelings are all okay.

43

Reach out to other moms who have experienced traumatic births and let them hear you out. Try joining support groups that can help you through your time as a NICU mom, if your baby is still in the hospital. Seek counseling if you feel like you cannot process your emotions with the help of your partner or your peers. There is incredible strength in being able to reach out and say, "I am not coping." Given the opportunity, spend as much time as you can with your baby, skin to skin, so that the two of you can bond outside of your home, or within your home. Don't be ashamed to be an advocate for yourself and for your baby, and, if you are feeling too exhausted, appoint someone to be an advocate for you both. If you are having thoughts of self-harming, harming your baby, or of complete detachment, reach out to a healthcare provider immediately. Often, the mixture of hormones and the fact that you have been through an incredibly traumatic event can trigger severe depression. Finally, try to be gentle with yourself and understand that you will heal and that, in time, you will bond with your baby, regardless of the type of birth you have had. Motherhood is by no means a sprint. It is a slow marathon that everyone runs at their own pace. You do not need to catch up with the next mom, you only need to ensure that you and your baby are the healthiest you can be.

Chapter 4: Feeding

Next to sleeping, your baby will spend most of their time nursing in the first few months of their life but you probably already knew that. What you may not know is that your baby will probably have a nursing personality and figuring out that personality through their cries and body language will probably happen around week four when the both of you have settled into a routine. Generally, your baby will fit into one of these five nursing types.

The Quick and Effective Feeder

Your little one will likely latch well and quickly, drinking their fill within 20 minutes. While this may be convenient from a time point of view, it may cause pain to breastfeeding moms. Making sure that your baby is latched correctly and switching breasts will help to ease the pain. For bottle-feeding moms, the quick effective feeder may cause themselves pain by ingesting too much wind, leading to excessive spit-up. To prevent this, break every five minutes during the feed to wind your baby, despite their protests.

Excitable Feeders

These little ones usually get excessively excited at the prospect of their next feed. They may not be able to latch correctly, or do not latch for long enough to get their fill. Bottle-fed babies may release the teat often, or dribble milk from the corners of their mouth. Both breast and bottle babies in this category will almost certainly begin fussing, crying, and eventually wind themselves up into a frustrating cycle of latching, unlatching, and screaming. Helping excitable feeders is thankfully very easy; offering their feed before they begin to gesture or fuss for milk will help to reduce excitement and being in a calm soothing environment will help to keep your baby relaxed. These types of feeders may be frustrating but are actually the easiest to get into a feeding routine.

The Sleeper

Your baby has shown all the signs of being hungry. They have latched like a champ and have begun drinking but, three minutes into the feed, they fall asleep. As a mom of a sleeper baby, you may feel like all you do is feed your baby, and you wouldn't be far from the truth. These little ones will demand to feed often as they are never getting their fill and will wake up after their feeding power nap unhappy that their stomach is not yet full. To get your sleeper to feed correctly, wake them to feed during the day and try to hold their attention during their feed. This can be done by gently brushing their cheek to stimulate the feeding reflex, massaging their feet, or talking to them. A little bit of persistence will get your little sleeper into a proper feeding routine quickly.

The Food Connoisseur

This little tyke will spend their time on their feed savoring every mouthful. These are your ideal feeders, taking time to drink slowly, negating wind to a large extent, and drinking to their fill. Food connoisseur feeders have the potential to become excitable feeders during growth spurts but will quickly return to their slow and steady self once the growth spurt has passed. There is no way to speed your little connoisseur up and you really shouldn't. Set aside 30 minutes per feed, regardless of what type of feeder you have, to ensure your baby has fed enough, is winded, and is ready to go down for their next nap with a full belly.

On / Off Feeder

Similar to the connoisseur feeder, on/off feeders do not like to be rushed. Typically, they will feed for a few minutes and rest for a few minutes. They may doze off like the sleeper but will quickly wake themselves to resume feeding. These little ones are extremely confusing for new moms as they are usually calm when no longer drinking and may seem that they have had their fill. As with the connoisseur, set aside a full 30 minutes to feed your little one so that you can be sure that they have had a full feed and that they are ready to be set down for their nap.

Breastfeeding

Breast or bottle? This is one of the most hotly debated topics among moms the world over. Deciding to breast or bottle-feed is an incredibly personal decision and ultimately will depend on the limitations of your lifestyle, medical conditions, and levels of comfort. Either way, your baby will be emotionally and nutritionally supported regardless of how you choose to feed them.

Having said that, the American Academy of Pediatrics suggests that a baby is exclusively breastfed for at least the first six months of their life and breastfeeding has its advantages. Aside from the financial aspect, a healthy mom provides the perfect balance of vitamins, minerals, and water to support a baby's growth, developmental and digestive needs. Breast milk is also packed with antibodies that prevent viral and bacterial illnesses. Emotionally, breastfeeding allows the perfect opportunity for skin-to-skin contact with your baby.

The most common questions asked by new breastfeeding moms is how many times a day will my baby eat and how do I know they are getting enough to eat? As we have mentioned before, each baby is different. Some may choose to nurse quickly and deeply until they take in their fill, while others may take their time, savoring every sip. Your newborn will need to nurse anywhere between eight and 12 times every 24 hours and will need between 10 and 15 minutes per breast in order to take in the nourishment they need. In the beginning, your baby will need to be breastfed on-demand which will be every one to three hours. No newborn should go more than four hours without a feed. As you demand feed your baby, a schedule will begin to be established, and eventually, you will both settle into a routine. Some moms are unsure as to when their baby is hungry and often, your baby will try to rush their feed or become frustrated as they try to satiate their hunger. Crying is the last sign of your baby's hunger and they will display some other signs before they begin to cry. These signs can be quick, but methodical movements of their head from side-to-side, opening their mouth and trying to suck any object close to them, sticking their tongue out, putting their hands or fists into their mouth, and pushing their head into your breasts. Your baby will go through growth spurts and their feeding schedule will change as they get older. Your newborn will need to feed for five to 10 minutes per breast per feed. In the first three days after your baby is born, your baby may only demand between four and seven feeds as their body acclimatizes to the outside world. These feeds will be rich with colostrum which is essential for your baby in the first few days and will help your milk to 'come in'. After this 'coming in' period, your baby may want to feed up to 12 times a day. Your breastfed newborn baby should never go more than three hours without a feed. From around day 30 of your baby's life, they will have settled into a nursing routine and will want to feed between 20 and 30 minutes per breast. This is just in time for their first big growth spurt at around Day 40 when they will, in all likelihood, want to cluster feed. This is when your little one demands smaller, more frequent feeds. By six weeks old, your baby will be feeding every three to four hours and may sleep for up to six hours a night. Breastfeeding does take a massive commitment from you, mom, but by month four, you and your baby should have established a good feeding and nighttime sleeping routine with your little one feeding five to six times per day and sleeping longer at night.

While we all want what is best for our baby, sometimes breastfeeding comes with limitations. Some new moms may need to return to work and will decide to express their feeds for their baby to bottle feed, while will have given birth to babies who require time in NICU. Certain health conditions and illnesses, such as HIV, and medications, like chemotherapy, prohibit moms from breastfeeding. If you are unsure of whether you can breastfeed due to medication or illness, if you would like to express for your baby, or if you are having issues with latching, contact your local breastfeeding support service to help you through your emotions and your decision-making process.

Bottle Feeding

Bottle-fed babies, like their breastfed counterparts, will need to be fed on demand for the first four weeks of their lives. This means your newborn will need to be fed every three to four hours. Formula-fed babies are more likely to sleep through a feed and because of this, you may need to institute a feeding routine where you dream feed or wake your baby to eat. Commercial formulas are specifically designed to nourish your little one and moms should not deviate from mixing the formula as directed. Unlike breast milk babies, formula does not require additional vitamin D as it is developed to have the exact nutritional content your baby needs. Formula and bottle feeding does come with their own set of challenges. Added iron content in formula can mean that your baby may suffer from constipation in the early stages of feeding, bottles need to be cleaned and sterilized after every feed and your baby may swallow more air than a breastfed baby, meaning more time will need to be spent winding and taking breaks during the feed to ensure that your baby does not spit up too much. Formula does, however, digest slower than breastmilk and because of this, your baby will need fewer feeds as they get older. Bottle feeding allows your partner to bond with your baby at feeding times and can mean that you have a break at night if you and your partner have a feeding schedule. Where your newborn will need to be bottle-fed every three to four hours, from two months this will extend to every four to five hours and after six months every five to six hours. Bottle-feeding requires preparation and organization to ensure that you are always on top of your baby's feeds. Imagine running out of formula, or not having enough milk expressed without your breast being readily available? You will need to be fastidious with cleaning bottles and teats and you will need to test each feed for the right temperature to ensure that you don't inadvertently burn your baby's mouth. Likewise, a bottle that is too cold will cause uncomfortable cramps and wind and bottles should be at room temperature, at the least to make it comfortable for your baby to drink. Never warm your baby's bottle in the microwave as it can cause hotspots because of the uneven heating process. Bottle feeding also comes with a fair amount of guesswork. Where breastfed babies will let their mom know they have had their fill, bottle-fed babies will often finish a feed and not demand more food. You will need to be aware of your baby's cues, looking out for signs that they are still hungry and will need to adjust their feed accordingly. The advantage of bottle feeding is that you will know exactly how much your baby has eaten in one feed and will be able to adjust their feed accordingly.

Is My Baby Eating Enough

If your baby is satisfied, not fussing, crying, or gesturing for a feed, chances are that they are getting enough to drink. If you are still concerned, keeping track of their diaper count can help to put your mind at rest. Your baby should produce between six and eight wet diapers per day. Breast milk babies will produce more soiled poop diapers than formula-fed babies as breast milk digests more easily. The most common concern for moms with feeding though is the amount that their baby spits up. While it is normal for your little one to bring up a little milk during feeding, large amounts of spit up can be a cause for concern. Allergies, digestive issues, reflux, and GERD (Gastrointestinal Reflux Disease), can cause your baby to spit up excessively. If your baby is not gaining weight steadily, seems dehydrated, not satiated after a feed, or does not have sufficient wet diapers you should contact your pediatrician or physician to ascertain if your baby requires a change in their diet or in your diet.

When your baby is born, their stomach is about the size of a marble. It will stretch and grow as your baby feeds more and begins to adjust to life outside of the womb. It is nearly impossible to know how much your baby has fed if you breastfeed and you will need to learn what your baby's hunger and satiation cues are and, eventually your own body's ability to increase feeds as your baby grows. A typical newborn bottle-fed baby will feed every two to four hours. How often they drink will depend on whether you have decided to formula or breast milk feed. It is important to remember that your breast milk baby will not necessarily drink more but will demand more frequent feeds because of the rate at which their body digests the milk.

Table 11. Feeding in Ounces/Milliliters

Age	Ounces/Milliliters	Solids & Water
0 to 2 weeks old	0.5 to 3 oz (14 to 90ml)	No
2 weeks to 2 months old	2 to 4 oz (60 to 120ml)	No
2 to 4 months old	4 to 6 oz (120 to 180ml)	No
4 to 6 months old	4 to 8oz (120 to 240ml)	Possibly
6 to 12 months old	8ox (240ml)	Yes

The Don'ts of Breastfeeding and Bottlefeeding

What would life be without a list of don't do that? Thankfully, the do not list for feeding your baby between birth and six months is not extensive.

Do not give your baby any liquid other than breastmilk or formula for the first six months of their life. This includes water, herbal teas, and any milk other than breast or formula. Liquids outside of mom's milk and scientifically developed formula will upset your baby's stomach, can cause constipation, reflux, indigestion, and will ultimately affect your baby's weight gain. Once your baby reaches six months and has begun their solid food journey you can offer some water between feeds but do not replace their milk intake as yet.

Do not add cereal to your baby's bottle in an attempt to thicken it or stretch feeds. Cereal is a choking hazard, and if your baby is not ready for solids, will pose a serious problem with their digestive system. If your baby has severe reflux opt to change out their formula for an anti-reflux brand or speak to your pediatrician about pediatric thickening agents.

Do not prop your baby's bottle next to them when they feed. While this may seem convenient, especially in the sleep-deprived early hours of the morning, feeding your baby like this can cause them to choke, aspirate their own spit-up, and will inevitably cause ear infections.

Do not sleep with your baby while you are breastfeeding. The risk of suffocation and rolling onto your baby as you sleep is very high.

Finally, do not expect your baby to fit into a perfect mold. Your little one will be unique in their feeding needs. Premature babies will need to have their ages adjusted until they have caught up at around 18 months old. Some babies eat more and some eat less. As long as your little one is picking up weight and feeding frequently, you are doing a great job of nourishing them.

The Scoop on Solids

Your baby may be ready to begin eating solids between the ages of four and six months. Breastfed babies may not need or want to start solids earlier than six months, and that is fine. Starting your baby on solids too early is not a great idea for your little one's digestive system. Their digestive enzymes may not be fully developed to move solids through their system. There are some telltale signs that your baby may be ready to begin eating though and if you follow their cues, you will be well on the way to a solid fed baby. These signs will present themselves in all babies. They include;

1. A firm neck and the ability to hold their head up when they are seated. A baby who cannot hold their head up will not be

able to swallow thicker consistencies and will choke if fed even pureed foods. You should not offer chunky food or follow baby-led weaning protocols until your baby is between seven and eight months old.

2. Your baby's tongue-thrust reflex will disappear. If you are not sure whether this reflex has gone, you can try and introduce some cereal mixed with breast or formula milk via a baby spoon. If your baby pushes the food out of their mouth after a few attempts, their tongue-thrust reflex is still in place and you will need to wait a little longer before introducing solids.

3. A keen interest in your food. You may notice that your little one has begun to show interest in your food. They may try to grab food from your hand, mimic you chewing and start trying to open your mouth as you put food into it. This is a sure sign that your baby is about ready to try solids.

4. Your baby has the ability to open their mouth wide and will gesture with an open mouth when food is presented.

Once your baby is showing all or most of these signs you can begin to introduce solids into their diet slowly. There is no right or wrong time of the day to introduce solids. For me, personally, the time of day when I was least rushed or preoccupied was best. Feeding your baby solids is the beginning of a messy and sometimes hilarious chapter in your lives together and should not be rushed. Thankfully, babies are really good and let us know when they are hungry, and when they are full. Watch your baby's cues and introduce solids when they are hungry but not starving to prevent accidental choking. Make sure that the baby is sitting upright, wide awake, and receptive, mouth open for the bite. You can try to put a little food on their fingers at first to get them accustomed to the texture and taste before introducing a baby spoon to their mouth. If they spit out the food but continue to ask for more, try again. It is not uncommon for babies to battle at first to get the hang of swallowing more solid textures. Don't worry about overfeeding, once your baby is full they will refuse to open their mouth or turn their head away from the spoon.

So what do you start your baby on when you are both ready to transition to solids?

Cereals are a good place to start as they have been specifically designed to be an easy introduction to the world of solids for your baby. Stick to brands that are tried, tested, and approved for use in babies and prepare it with breast or formula milk. Do not introduce cow's milk to your baby's diet until they are a year old. Cereal should initially be a soup-like consistency and can be thickened gradually as they become used to the taste and texture. Once your baby has become accustomed to cereal you can begin to introduce pureed yellow or orange vegetables like sweet potatoes and carrots. Try to keep tastes bland and do not add salt or sugar to your purees. If your baby rejects vegetables to start with, try again. Most little ones can take up to 15 attempts before they become used to a new taste or texture. Pureed fruits like apples, pears and avocado can be introduced once your baby is used to vegetables. Be aware that bananas, while easy to mash, can be difficult to digest and may cause severe constipation. Meats, eggs, pasta, beans, tofu, and whole cheeses and yogurts should only be introduced after seven months and one at a time to allow your baby's digestive system time to adjust. From around eight months, you can try to introduce baby-led weaning, which isa system in which your baby begins to eat small bite-sized soft items that are not pureed.

As with breast and formula feeding, there are some solid don'ts.

Don't introduce your baby to foods that are easy choking hazards. These include peas, nuts, grapes, hotdogs, or anything that is not cut into small sizes and cannot be squashed with gentle pressure between your fingers.

Avoid high allergen foods like nuts, eggs, cows milk, fish, shellfish, and wheat.

Don't leave your baby unattended with their food. Choking can happen quickly and unexpectedly.

Don't panic if your baby gags. Learn the difference between choking and gagging and take a first aid course so that you know what to do if your baby does choke.

Food Allergies

The jury is still out on whether delaying the introduction of common allergy foods prevents allergic attacks. You will need to use your discretion and know your family history of allergies should you wish to introduce these foods earlier rather than later. Most children will grow out of food allergies by the time they are five years old but some will have specific allergies for life. Allergic signs can range from moderate to severe and will need different courses of action depending on the reaction. Gassiness, diarrhea, excess mucus, and mild vomiting can be corrected by avoiding the food that caused them whereas more severe reactions like a rash, hives, a swollen mouth, excessive itching, and difficulty breathing should warrant a visit to the emergency room. Foods that cause severe reactions should be avoided entirely until your baby is at least five years old.

Common allergy goods that should be avoided until your baby is at least eight months old include; cow's milk, eggs, gluten or wheat products, nuts and peanuts, seeds including sesame and poppy seeds, soy, shellfish, fish, preservatives and food colorings, some citrus and strawberries. If your baby shows signs of being allergic to any of the above foods, you will need to read labels carefully to avoid triggers.

While processed meats, honey, chicken, and deli meats may not be classified as high allergen foods, they should be avoided for the first year of your baby's life. This is because these products contain bacteria that your baby's immune system cannot fight as yet and may make your baby incredibly ill.

Establishing a good eating regime with your baby will be half the battle won when it comes to becoming routined together. The next step in your routine journey will be establishing a sleep schedule that works for you both.

Chapter 5: Sleeping

Babies sleep a lot! Your newborn will sleep between 14 and 17 hours per day. Sleeping like a baby makes more sense now. Doesn't it? While your baby may sleep an exorbitant amount of time, their feeding schedule and need to eat around the clock often makes that sleep sporadic and restless. In the beginning, your baby will be awake for between 30 minutes and an hour at a time and can sleep for between 15 minutes and three hours. Newborns will demand a feed when they wake but will not spend much time awake. As your baby grows, their sleeping time will become less and less as they take in the world around them and demand more stimulation. Sleep is incredibly important for your baby as this is when they grow, learn, and develop.

As you establish your feeding routine, sleeping patterns should begin to develop as well but this is not always the case. Newborns can't tell the time and since they have spent 9 months in total darkness, they may confuse day and night. This usually corrects itself but some tips and tricks can be learned to help ease your little one into daylight hour routines that don't involve you being awake all night. Perhaps the most important thing to take away from this chapter is that well-rested moms have well-rested babies. Studies have shown that your baby will pick up on your frustration, and aggravation and can lead to your baby mimicking your feelings, making it harder for you to calm your baby into a sleepy state. Seasoned moms will tell you that the world will not come to an end if your home is not 100% clean, or if you skip a shower day. Getting a 30-minute nap in with your baby, and taking care of yourself is far more important than conforming to an expectation to be perfect all of the time.

Basic Sleep Principles

As we mentioned before, your baby will start their lives with between 14 and 17 hours of sleep a day. Some babies may even stretch that to 18 or 19 hours while they are going through a growth spurt. It is important that you do not allow your baby to skip a feed, especially in the beginning phases of their life. This means that you will need to feed your baby every two to three hours if you are a breastfeeding mom and every three to four hours if you are formula feeding. Your baby's stomach is not big enough just yet to go without a feed and choosing to let your baby sleep can lead to serious health issues. If your baby does not wake during daylight hours to feed, you can gently wake them to ensure that they do feed. At night, you can institute a dream feeding routine to keep your baby in a sleepy state while they feed. As your baby gets older, they will begin to sleep for a longer period at night, stretching to between five and six hours from around three months of age. Remember that every baby is different though. My first baby would never sleep for longer than two hours, even through the night, and eventually, we all had a full night's rest just after his second birthday. My subsequent babies enjoyed their sleep and were dream-fed from day one to allow them to rest through the night.

Most moms will decide to room-share with their baby until they are slightly older. Whether you choose to have your baby sleep in a crib, bassinet, or co-sleeping crib is entirely up to you. Bed-sharing is not recommended due to the increased risk of accidental smothering and Sudden Infant Death Syndrome. If you do choose to have your baby sleep in their own nursery from early on, a good breathing and baby monitor should be bought and you should have a quiet, comfortable spot set up in the nursery to feed so that you are not waking your baby for nighttime feeds. Your baby's crib or bassinet should have an approved, breathable mattress, an approved mattress protector, and a tightly fitted baby approved sheet. The crib or bassinet needs to be free of any toys, pillows, blankets, comforter, crib bumpers, plushies, or non fitted sheets. When putting your baby down to sleep, place them on their back, you can alternate which side their head faces to prevent their head from taking on a strange shape, and to avoid neck stiffness. By three months, your baby will be able to move their head from side to side themselves. Do not prop their head up so that it is facing the ceiling. Your baby may spit-up and if their head is to the side, this will pour out of their mouth freely. Your baby should sleep in a room that is clean and free of dust, cigarette smoke, and perfume. If your little one enjoys a pacifier but spits it out once asleep, don't force it back into their mouth. For information on what your baby should sleep in, how many layers are required, and what blankets and swaddles to purchase, consult our 'Shopping for Baby' chapter.

While trying to find a sleep routine may be a little difficult in the beginning, reading the signs of sleepiness in your baby is easy when you know what you are looking for. Your little one may be fussy but will have been fed and changed, may be reluctant to make eye contact, and will look away from you, rub their eyes, and yawn often. These are all signs that your baby is ready for a nap. Try and put your baby in their crib or bassinet when they are sleepy but still awake as this gives your baby a positive association with their sleep area and signals them to sleep. The urge to cuddle and rock your baby to sleep will be difficult to resist in the beginning, and there is nothing wrong with the occasional snuggle to sleep but remember that your baby will grow quickly, and rocking, walking, and hushing a bigger baby is not easy, nor is breaking bad sleeping habits. Learning how to fall asleep with mom close by and the usual sounds of the house in the background will be the single most valuable lesson you will teach your baby initially and will save you a whole lot of time and tears later in your baby's life.

Once your baby is asleep, you may find yourself watching them, marveling at the cuteness you have brought into this world, and watching their every breath. Watching your baby sleep can bring hours of endless entertainment but may also have you wondering if the faces they are pulling, strange sounds, and odd eye movements are normal. Newborn babies are incredibly restless sleepers and may squirm, wake suddenly before drifting off again and spend a huge chunk of their sleeping time in the REM (rapid eye movement) stage. While they are in this phase, they may whimper, smile, or even cry out, which brings us to the weird and wonderful noises a sleeping baby makes. Baby's breath at a rate of 40 to 60 breaths per minute while they are awake but that may slow down to between 30 and 40 breaths per minute while they sleep. Some babies will take slow breaths, skip a breath, or may take a series of rapid breaths for around 20 seconds before pausing their breathing for a few seconds. While this may freak you out as a new mom, it is completely normal. Their little brain has not quite learned how to regulate breathing as yet and as your baby sleeps and grows, this center will begin to function more efficiently. If you are concerned about your baby's breathing patterns, baby monitoring sleep mats can be bought to alert you of a problem with your baby's breathing and will allow you some information to provide your pediatrician with if you choose to consult them on your baby's breathing. Some of the noises your baby makes while breathing include rattling, whistling, and strange but normal gurgling sounds. While these may be alarming at first, you will become accustomed to them as your new normal night sounds. If your baby is breathing rapidly, more than 70 breaths a minute for an extended period of time, grunts with every exhale, have nostrils that are flaring, or the muscles under their ribs are pulling in or contracting, contact your doctor or visit your emergency room immediately, as these are all signs of respiratory distress.

Sleep Newborn to Three Months

At this stage, you're probably going to feel like you are in a constant cycle of eat-sleep- poop and repeat. Moms will often find the newborn to three-month phase to be the most exhausting, even if your little one isn't awake for most of the day. Often termed the 'sleep survival' stage, newborn to three months is the perfect time to institute a good relationship with sleep for you and your bundle of joy. At this age, your baby will sleep between 14 and 17 hours during a 24 hour period but this may vary between 11 and 19 hours, depending on growth spurts and your little one's own sleep needs. Your baby may sleep anywhere from 30 minutes to hours hours per nap time and will need round the clock feeds. Because of this, it is important that you get the rest you need and deserve as well. In this phase, it will be unlikely that you will be able to institute a sleep routine as your baby has an enormous amount of growing to do and their feeding schedule simply won't permit proper routines to be put into place but setting your little one up with a good sleep relationship is vital at this point.

Remember that your newborn spends 9 months in darkness and because of this, may need a little extra help in falling asleep during the day. Drawing the curtains and making sure that their sleep environment is calm will help your baby understand that daytime is also time. During this phase of your baby's life, you may swaddle them to help them feel safe and secure but once your baby can roll, or has passed the three month mark, swaddling is no longer recommended as they may roll over in the middle of a nap and be unable to roll back. As your baby grows through their first three months, nighttime sleep will stretch to around four or five hours and they will sleep for longer periods of time during the day between feeds. It is important to not allow your baby to sleep for too long of a stretch during the day as they may confuse day and night leading to frustrating all-night conversations with your awake little angel. The good news is that developing a healthy sleeping pattern at this age is pretty easy if you watch for your baby's sleep cues. Missing these cues at this age though can be disastrous, with your baby becoming overstimulated. A hysterical baby who seems more alert, overactive, has glazed looking eyes, and cries easily is very difficult to get to sleep and will need a little extra effort to calm.

Most importantly, be patient with yourself at this phase of your journey into motherhood. There are going to be times where you are so thoroughly exhausted that you feel like you cannot possibly do anything other than sleep with your baby and that is absolutely fine. Sleeping during the day, napping with your little one after a feed, and spending some downtime doing absolutely nothing before the next feed and poop will go a long way in helping you to feel a little less exhausted.

Sleep Three Months to Six Months

Aaah! Blissful sleep! By three months, your baby will begin to sleep around five hours per night and by six months they may be sleeping a full eight hours. This is not to say that all babies begin sleeping through but most will only wake once a night. From three months, daytime naps will be less frequent but will probably be longer with the normal range being one to two hours per daytime nap. By this time, your baby should have established a healthy relationship with sleep and will be ready to begin sleep training if you choose to do so. Babies three months and older should not be swaddled anymore and should have graduated to a sleep sack or bag. On average, your three month old will sleep between 10 and 18 hours in a 24 hour period with between two and three daytime naps. They will have less active sleep cycles and will begin to settle into quiet sleep which is the way adults sleep.

While this might all sound incredible for you poor sleep-deprived moms, you may hit a snag. Your baby's sleep pattern is ever-changing and because they are due a large developmental growth spurt around four months old, sleep regression may occur. Now before you panic! Sleep regression can be beaten, and relatively easily at that if you have established a good sleep relationship. This regression happens not only because of their growth spurt but because your baby is easing into adult sleep patterns and has suddenly become incredibly conscious of the world around them. This means that they are consciously aware of the fact that they are drifting off to sleep and may end up fighting it. Because of this, it is important for you to provide a calm environment that facilitates sleep and institute a routine and sleep ritual that works for you both. If you have been rocking your baby to sleep, they will expect it to continue as they now associate the comfort of mom's arms with drifting off. This could mean that you spend the better part of your day trying to replicate the sleep relationship rituals you instituted before three months. The big difference now is that your baby will realize that you have put them down during their light sleep cycle and will insist that you pick them up to repeat the process. If you have chosen not to put your baby down to sleep,it will take some time and patience to help them relearn a healthy sleep pattern. Sleep regression unfortunately does not go away by itself and you will need to teach your baby to self settle for them to develop a healthy sleeping pattern. At this age, sleep is as important as nutrition to your little one's development. Too little daytime sleep is going to mean a miserable baby who won't settle at night and will probably revert back to their newborn waking routine.

Creating Good Sleeping Habits

You now know how much sleep your baby needs and why they need it as well as the importance of a good sleep relationship. Creating that sleep relationship for your baby can be a very personal journey, and aside from feeding, can be one of the greatest bonding experiences you have with your little one. Following some of these tips and tricks may help you to decode what works for your baby in creating a good sleep relationship and, ultimately, a nap and sleep schedule that works well for both of you.

Your newborn baby will need to be exposed to consistent cues on when to sleep. Because of their inability to tell day from night, they will need time to sync with light and dark schedules. When you give your newborn strong, consistent cues, such as routined feeding, diaper changing, and swaddling before you put them down to sleep, you are allowing them to understand that these actions trigger sleep. During their waking daylight hours, expose them to the hustle and bustle of your home so that they can differentiate between calm sleep and normal life. For nighttime sleep, try not to expose your baby to too much light. Opt for soft lighting that doesn't trigger their waking response. Don't be overly aware of diaper changing. If your baby's diaper is not full or they have not poop soiled it, chances are you can skip one nighttime change.

Make sure that your little one is calm and feels secure before you put them down to sleep regardless of the time of day. As exhausted as you are, your stress and irritation will ultimately upset your baby and the two of you will feed off of each other. Do not worry about taking a time out when you feel that the two of you are feeding off of each other's frustration. Pass your baby onto your partner or, if you are alone with the baby, stop trying to make them sleep. Instead, take a walk together to break the pattern of frustration and try again in a few minutes. If you feel that your baby is overstimulated, you can try baby wrapping them to your chest until they drift off to sleep.

Babies who are not sleepy will not sleep. You cannot force your little one to sleep if they are not ready. Watch for their sleep cues and wind them down for their nap or bedtime by removing them from external stimulants like noisy spaces, and televisions. Keep sleep time noise ambient and, if at all possible, take some quiet time for yourself. Try not to allow your baby to take long late afternoon naps as these can often lead to frustratingly long evenings of trying to get your little one settled and confused sleep schedules. If your baby does accidentally sleep too long and too late in the afternoon, keep them up a little later than usual, watch for their sleep cues and then let them have a longer than usual feed before putting them down to sleep. At night don't be too enthusiastic about jumping out of bed to see them. Remember that babies are noisy sleepers and will go through periods of light sleep in which they can appear as if they are awake. Instead, leave your baby until you are sure they are fussing for a feed during the night and avoid stimulating them with conversation, eye contact, or light. When your baby is old enough, around four months, you can try and institute a once a night dream feed in which you do not wake them but rather feed and put them straight back down to sleep. This may help your little one to stretch their nighttime sleep for a full five to eight hours.

Sometimes, there is absolutely nothing you can do to console your baby or help them to sleep. Infant colic, severe reflux, and certain sleep conditions can hinder your baby's sleep patterns and cause them distress before they are even put down to sleep. Speaking to your pediatrician may help to come up with medical solutions while reaching out to other moms will help with more practical support. If your baby suffers from any sleep issues that are depriving you both of much-needed sleep, reach out to those you can trust to look after your little one while you catch up on some sleep. Colic and reflux may feel like they will last forever but it will eventually subside and you will both get the sleep you need. In the meantime, a few daytime naps while your baby is being taken care of will allow you to have some downtime and recuperate.

Sleep Troubleshooting

You may feel like you have tried absolutely everything to get your little one to sleep and sometimes you would be right. There are times when your baby will have reasons why they are not sleeping and while sleep disorders do happen in babies, they are rare. Sleep regression, growth spurts, and overstimulation can all lead to your baby battling to sleep but going through our handy troubleshooting guide should help you to find some solutions to your angel's insistence on being awake.

My baby sleeps longer and more peacefully during the day.

Chances are your baby has confused day and night. Fixing day/night confusion is relatively easy. Exposing your baby to daytime activities and sunlight, avoiding nighttime sleep routines during the day, and keeping your baby awake a little longer during their daytime wake period will help to rectify time confusion quickly.

My baby is not giving sleep cues at their bedtime.

Babies can be trained to sleep around certain times of day but will not always conform to exact times. Chances are that your little one has confused day and night and, by following the steps above, you will be able to reset their internal clock. By three months old, they will have begun to develop light sleep cycles and will begin to consciously accept sleep as a positive part of their lives.

Why is my baby fussing and moving their head from side to side at sleep time?

Chances are your baby is hungry or is looking for a top-up comfort feed. Some babies like to tank feed before nighttime sleep and this will mean that you may need to feed a little longer for them to settle in for the night.

My baby's eyes are glassy, they are showing sleep cues but will not settle.

Your little one is probably overstimulated and needs time to wind down. Try to remove them from noise, light, and external stimulants and swaddle or soothe them until they calm. If your baby still won't calm, try to baby wrap them to yourself as a temporary fix. Once they have drifted off to sleep, place them in their crib.

Why won't my baby go to sleep at a consistent time?

It could be that a good sleep routine has not been established. Babies thrive on routine and although they will not adhere strictly to your times, a roundabout routine time to sleep will give your baby a sense of order and will help them to understand when they are meant to sleep.

Why does my baby wake at 4 a.m. to start the day?

There are several reasons why your baby could be starting their day too early. A bedtime that is too early, or too late can cause issues in sleep patterns and may have your baby waking early in the morning to start their day. Other times, parents are too quick to intervene when they hear their baby stirring. Between 4 and 5 a.m. is the most likely time for your baby to wake; responding too quickly or with too much stimulation will have your baby roused into a fully awake state.

My baby doesn't settle quickly after nighttime feeds.

I know the urge to have a conversation with your angel at night can be overwhelming but try and keep night feed stimulation to an absolute minimum. Keep your lights dimmed, avoid eye contact and diaper changes and don't talk to your little one.

My baby is inconsolable and this is a new thing.

If your baby is suddenly inconsolable, cries when put down, and seems generally uncomfortable, they may not feel well. The most common culprit for an uncomfortable baby is gas. Try winding your little one patiently working each stuck gas bubble out. If they are still crying when you put them down, they may have an earache or ear infection and will need to be seen by a pediatrician or physician. If your baby is pulling their legs up and hasn't had a soiled poop diaper in more than 24 hours, they may be constipated and will need laxative relief. From as early as six weeks, drooling, fist biting and clenching of the jaw may be an indication that your baby is teething and may need medication to relieve their discomfort.

The 5 S's of Sleeping

There will be times where your little one will be fussy and may need a little extra help to soothe. Harvey Karp, a pediatrician, is a pioneer in soothing methods and developed the five S's method to help moms when their baby is constantly fussy. These S's stand for swaddle, side-stomach position, shush, swing and suck, and have been shown to be incredibly effective in calming and soothing fussy, crying, and overstimulated babies. Sometimes no amount of playing, feeding, winding, and diaper changing can get your baby to settle and that is when the five s's come into play.

The five s's should be followed in this order;

Swaddle

Learning how to swaddle your baby properly is one of the most valuable lessons you will learn for the early weeks of their lives. After being wrapped up all snuggly in your womb for nine months, swaddling reminds them of those days. It also prevents your baby's startle reflex which some baby's deploy to wake themselves.

Side-Stomach Position

There has been a lot of research done on the optimal position for your baby to sleep. This research shows that babies who sleep on their stomach generally sleep for longer and have less startle reaction to wake them. But, as we have mentioned, stomach sleeping is incredibly dangerous and increases the risk of SIDS. The solution? Holding your baby on their stomach, side, over your shoulder, or on your forearm supporting their head with your hand. Once your baby has calmed, you can put them down in their crib or bassinet on their back as usual.

Shush

You may think that your baby spent nine months in your womb softly cushioned away from noise. This is not entirely true. The gurgling of your stomach, muffled outside noises, and the sound of your blood pumping through your body are all sounds they heard while nestled inside you. By making a loud shhh sound while continuing to introduce them to the muted sounds of your house, you are pretty close to mimicking the sounds they are used to. This comforts your baby and makes them feel like they are safely tucked back in your womb.

Swing

A soft swinging motion is an excellent way to get your baby to soothe and calm down. Research has shown that gently swinging or rocking your baby lowers their heart rate and communicates to them that it is time to sleep. Movements should be kept small and their neck and head should be supported at all times. Never, ever shake your baby or swing them violently.

Suck

Sucking is one of your baby's primitive reflexes. They practiced it in the womb and know that sucking will ultimately lead to nourishment and soothing. Some moms may choose to offer their breast to suck on while others will offer a pacifier in order to soothe their little one. Don't worry about your baby becoming dependent on a pacifier or thumb. Your baby is not capable of forming bad habits until they are six months old.

When you use the five s's method you are likely to bond with your baby while helping them to soothe and transition into sleep.

Chapter 6: Caring For Your Newborn

Beyond feeding and changing your baby, taking time to bond with your little one will help you to better understand their needs. Bonding is usually a natural process for some moms but others, the process can take a little longer. Rest assured that your feelings of detachment will disappear and if it does not, you may be suffering from postpartum depression and will need to see your physician. Your baby is pre-programmed to initiate a relationship with you. Their cries, noise, smiles, breast searching, and insistence of eye contact are all ways in which they communicate their bond with you and form a meaningful attachment.

Sometimes these initial attachments cannot happen. Moms and babies are separated at birth when a baby requires NICU or the mom requires special or specific care. This can lead to feelings of separation anxiety for your little one and may lead to new moms into depression or feelings of inadequacy. Fortunately, most separations are temporary and these early bonding opportunities can be simulated to create a natural attachment. This is why parents can adopt and still have a wonderful relationship with their child. Remember to include the other parent in the bonding process to allow for your baby to feel safe and secure with all of their primary caregivers.

Contrary to popular belief, you cannot spoil your baby in their early days. Bad habits and non-routine habit-forming only occur after six months of age. Failure to bond with your baby can be severely detrimental to your little one's emotional and physical development. Because of this, it is important for you to spend a sufficient amount of time to bond adequately, learning what their cues are, reading their crying language, and understanding the signs they are giving you. This will all allow you to bond well with your little one.

Bonding With Your Baby

Your baby will attempt to bond with you naturally. This is done with specific natural instincts they have been equipped with to ensure their survival while they are at their most vulnerable stage of their life. For some moms, natural bonding is either interrupted or does not come naturally, but there are ways to encourage bonding between mom and baby which will speed along your natural bonding process and allow you to develop a good relationship with your baby.

Regular Touch

Your baby has spent nine months curled up warm and snug in the womb. Being born into a world of noise and light can be overwhelming and your baby will be looking to feel secure and safe. These feelings of safety allow your newborn time to make eye contact with you and to portray their own needs through facial expressions, crying, and gesturing while helping them to calm their startle reflex.

Learn Their Cry Language

Babies cry for a reason and these cries should be responded to as quickly as possible and appropriately. If you aren't sure why your baby is crying, go through the process of feeding, winding, changing, swaddling. You can employ the five S's to try and soothe your little one. Ignoring your baby's cries for extended periods of time can lead to feelings of abandonment and will leave your baby feeling unsafe.

Spend Time Holding Them

Premature babies who have skin on skin contact have been shown to grow and heal quicker than babies who are not permitted to have skin contact. Holding, rocking, and spending time skin on skin will help to bond with your baby. As your baby grows, you can carry them in a sling or baby wrap to encourage bonding while getting things done around the home. This is not to say that you will not need to encourage quiet time together but baby wrapping is a convenient way to keep your baby safe and secure.

Create Physical Safety

Your newborn will need to feel physically safe. Swaddling, providing good neck and head support while you hold your baby. When your baby does not feel safe, their brain will produce cortisol, a stress hormone that will prevent them from settling and bonding with you.

Use All Forms of Communication

As adults, we use a series of facial expressions, hand gestures, and spoken language to communicate our needs. Your baby already knows the sounds you make from spending time in your womb but will need to learn other forms of soothing communication. Make eye contact with your baby and speak to them in soothing tones, tell them stories, and sing them songs. You will be surprised at just how well normal adult communication works on calming your baby and facilitates the natural bond between you.

Baby Interaction

Baby's communicate their needs through various cues. We have already gone through their sleepy and hungry cues but did you know that your little one can tell you when they want to play, when they are scared and when they are content? Learning to read these cues is important for you and your baby, especially when they seem to be stuck in an endless loop of frustrating crying. When you know what your baby wants, it makes it so much easier to understand the cause of their crying and, let's face it, babies under the age of six months cry a lot!

Signs that your baby is alert and ready interact with you include normal, pink skin color, arms, and legs that flex and tuck rhythmically, bringing their hand to their mouth but not sucking it, or touching their face, trying to focus on their balled fists, pursing their lips, beautiful gummy smiles that include eye contact, and relaxed, happy sounds. When your little ones display some, of, or all of these cues, they are communicating to you that they are ready to play and spend some time bonding with you. As your baby grows, you will be able to hold their attention for more and more time, but initially, they will become overstimulated or tired pretty quickly. Signs that they have had enough activity for the moment include sleep cues, hiccupping, sneezing, refusal to make eye contact or looking away from you, frantic leg and arm movements, and of course crying. Finding the balance between how much is enough interaction between the two of you will not take long, and if your baby does become overstimulated occasionally, don't worry about it. By following the tips and tricks we've already provided, you should be able to calm your little one. Some of these physical interactions are rooted in primal reflexes and are designed to let moms know what babies need or are trying to communicate at a primal level.

The Moro Reflex

Also called the startle reflex, your baby will respond to anything that scares them by flailing their arms and/or legs and clenching their fists. This reflex is in place from the time your baby is born and will generally disappear between four and six months. This cue lets you know that something has frightened your baby and is their first attempt to protect themselves. If your baby's Moro reflex startles them awake often, you can try swaddling them. Should your baby not have the Moro reflex, please contact your pediatrician to have your baby assessed for nerve injury or sore limbs.

Rooting Reflex

Remember when we told you about your little one's insistence on sucking when you touch their cheek? This is called the rooting reflex and is your baby's way of telling you they are hungry. Your baby's rooting reflex will last until they are about four months old but they may continue to suck in their sleep well into their toddler years. Premature babies may not have their rooting reflex as yet but, with a little patience and time, they will catch up and will be gesturing to suck when they are hungry.

Palmers Reflex

Also known as the grasp reflex, Palmers reflex is the one that tugs at almost everyone's heart. From birth, your baby will wrap their tiny fingers around anything that touches their hand but may, in the early days, also make them curl their toes up. While this reflex doesn't serve much of a purpose, to begin with, it does prepare them to be able to grasp onto things voluntarily later in their lives. The grasp reflex usually disappears at around six months of age or when your baby can consciously navigate the outside world and begin to grab onto things they want. If your baby is grasping you tightly, they may be signaling that they are feeling a little insecure and may need a cuddle.

Sucking Reflex

Different from your baby's rooting reflex, the sucking reflex is developed in the womb when they begin sucking their thumbs. Where the rooting reflex encourages your baby to find the source of their next feed and to signal they are hungry, the sucking reflex ensures that your baby can suck hard enough to drink. As with the rooting reflex, premature babies are often born with a poor sucking reflex but with a little bit of practice are able to catch up. This reflex generally disappears around four months old when your baby is consciously aware of the breast or bottle. If your baby begins sucking and gets frustrated, it's a sure sign that they are hungry.

The Crying Game

I've said it before and I will say it again, baby's cry a lot! The good news is that by month three, your little one should only be crying between one and two hours per day and these cries will be an indication that they need something or are generally uncomfortable. To begin with, though, your newborn will probably cry more than they don't. Fortunately, a baby's cries are a form of communication and almost every cry can be interpreted to mean something. While it will be up to you to decode what each cry means, generally every specific cry or niggle will signal what they need from you. A crying baby is thoroughly overwhelming for a new mom, but try to remain calm and watch your baby's cues to ascertain what they are crying for. Rooting and sucking along with crying signals they are hungry, even if you only fed them a short while ago. Side to side head movements, frantically shaking their arms and legs, and refusing eye contact while being inconsolable will mean they are overtired and need to be soothed to sleep. Dealing with your crying baby will become part of your life for a little while and you will need to learn some coping mechanisms to get through this phase of your little one's life.

Try and stay calm as you tune into your baby's mood and watch for their cues. Do not raise your voice or become frustrated with your little one as they will pick up on your mood and the situation will only escalate. If you feel like you cannot cope, call your partner or someone to help you while you and your little one calm down. If your baby has regular bouts of crying, try and keep a diary of the time of day and what worked to soothe them. Chances are that they may dislike a certain sound or smell in your home at that specific time and are protesting or they may be experiencing some form of colic discomfort. Trust your instincts! Even if your baby is giving cues that they need their diaper changed but you know they are due a feed and probably hungry, offer them a feed. Sometimes babies get confused and like adults, just feel otherwise and aren't entirely sure what they want at all. Be flexible in your approach to dealing with your crying baby. You may not feel like rocking them right this second but if that is what they want then that is what you are going to give them to get your baby to calm down. Remember, babies cannot get spoiled and are not capable of learning bad habits before three months of age. Finally, don't be embarrassed or ashamed to ask for help. Trust your gut above all things! If you feel there is something wrong with your baby, chances are that you are right. Babies will often cry or display discomfort before they show symptoms of being sick. If your baby is fussing constantly, will not settle, and is crying every time you put them down, get to your pediatrician or the emergency room to have your baby examined.

General Care

As a new mom, you will probably be inundated with information on what to do and what not to do when taking care of your baby. For some moms, generally, baby care classes can be taken before birth while others have mom friends or their own moms to help them in the early days after bringing your baby home. If you are one of those moms who hasn't had the chance to attend classes, or if your own mom isn't on hand to help you out, this book is here to help you with some of the general care issues new moms face.

Cord Care

Once you have come home with your baby, you will need to take care of their umbilical cord until it shrivels and falls off around Day 10. A baby's umbilical cord is probably one of the most amazing reminders that your baby was once attached to you and that you were able to nourish and grow them for nine months. Once your baby is born, the cord will be clamped and cut and a small portion of it will still be attached to your baby. This is called the stump and it will need to be cleaned. Usually, the stump will remain attached to your baby for between seven and 14 days and, during this time, it will be your responsibility to keep it clean and free of irritation. Pediatricians and midwives suggest using surgical spirits or a saltwater solution to keep your baby's stump clean while others suggest to only use water unless the stump gets pee or poop on it. The best time to clean your little one's stump is during their diaper change. You will need to make sure your hands are clean and dry. After removing the diaper, and before you close the next clean diaper up, gently move the cord from one side to the next while applying a little cleaning solution to the base of the stump where the cord and belly button meet. After bath time, do not clean your baby's stump but make sure that it is properly dried but gently patting it with a towel. When doing up your baby's diaper, try to fold down the front of the diaper so that it does not irritate the stump, and where possible, avoid putting your little one in pants until the stump has fallen off and the belly button has healed. Never try to pull your baby's stump off, even if it is hanging on by a thread! It will fall off in its own time and, if it has not detached after two weeks, you will need to take your baby to the doctor to have it seen to. Should the stump smell bad, be warm to the touch, or if the belly button has redness or inflammation around it, consult your pediatrician immediately as these are all signs of infection.

Once your baby's cord has fallen off, you are worried about the appearance of their belly button. As your baby grows, their belly button will change. If you suspect that your baby has a hernia or granuloma, a small red or pink lump in the belly button area, you can chat with your family physician. Most of the time, these conditions rectify themselves and are not anything to be concerned about.

Bathing Your Baby

Bathing your baby is a special time that can be used to create a bond with your baby. Most babies love the feeling of water but some will protest to begin with. Don't worry, most babies will eventually love their bathing time. Your baby will probably get their first bath in the hospital before you are both discharged, but if you have chosen home birth you may be wondering when your baby should get their first bath? The World Health Organization recommends that babies are not bathed for at least 24 hours after birth. This is because your baby is still adjusting to the outside world and may have trouble maintaining their body temperature. The vernix, (that strange waxy substance on your baby's skin directly after birth), is specifically designed to protect your little one's skin from the harsh outside world. Delaying their first bath will help to keep the skin moisturized and protected from external bacteria while their immune system begins to kick in within the first 24 hours.

How often your baby is bathed is entirely up to you but it is not necessary to bathe your baby every day. Babies rarely sweat enough in the first three months of their life to warrant daily baths and if they are particularly sweaty, you can opt to top and tail them rather than giving them a full bath. Many pediatricians still recommend that babies with their umbilical stump still attached are only sponge bathed to prevent the introduction of bacteria into the stump wound.

To sponge bath your baby, fill a portable basin or bucket with warm, temperate water. The water should neither feel too warm, nor too cool on your wrist. Lay your baby on a comfortable, flat surface like your bed, changing area, or sturdy counter near your sink but make sure that non-padded surfaces are soft. Ensure that your baby's towel is down before you begin sponge bathing them. Always use safety straps or keep your hand on your baby once they are on the bathing surface to prevent them from falling. Dip a washcloth, or cotton pad into the water, being sure to ring out excess water, and begin by washing your baby's face. Be careful not to get water in your baby's eyes, nose, or mouth. You will need to dip the cloth back into the water or get a new cotton pad to wash the remainder of your baby's body. Take special care to get into all of the folds and creases to get rid of accumulated dirt and prevent yeast infections. This is especially true for your little girl's vagina but never wash inside her vagina. Make sure that your baby remains covered with a towel or blanket through the sponge bathing process, only exposing the areas that are being washed. For the first two weeks of your baby's life, it will not be necessary to expose them to soap or other bath products to keep them clean.

Once your baby's stump has fallen off and the umbilical area has healed, you can introduce them to the tub or portable baby bath. It is important to never leave your baby alone in or around water. They may protest at first but, eventually, they will come to love water and if your baby becomes hysterical you can always go back to sponge bathing until they are ready for a normal bath. Make sure that, when you wash your baby's hair, their neck is well supported and that you never immerse your baby's head completely. From around four weeks of age, you can begin to introduce top and tail soaps or specifically designed baby washing products. If your baby shows signs of dry skin or eczema, ditch the product and go back to plain water. When removing your baby from the bath, make sure they go straight into a towel and get them dressed as quickly as possible. Most of all, have fun, keep your baby feeling safe, and remember water safety rules when bathing your baby.

Straight after your baby has had a bath as they drift off to sleep is the ideal time to clip your baby's nails. Your baby will be quiet, relaxed, and unaware of what you are doing. Make sure to use baby approved nail clippers, scissors, or a baby emery board to keep your baby's nails short, otherwise, you could choose to bite your baby's nails off rather than cutting them. If you are incredibly nervous about cutting your baby's nails, consult your local baby wellness clinic; they may cut them for you.

The Scoop on Poop

As a mom you're going to spend a whole lot of time talking about, changing, and examining your baby's poop. From black and tarry when they are first born to mustard color and grainy, when you wonder how their poop could possibly look like your little one ate mustard. Your baby's poop is an invaluable source of information when seeing if they are healthy.

When your baby is first born, they will probably only have one or two poops a day as they begin to increase their feeds and their digestive system adjusts to outside nourishment. By the end of your little one's first week outside of the womb, they will have between five and ten soiled poop diapers per day, although it is not uncommon for breastfed babies to poop after every feed. By week four, your baby's digestive system will begin to mature and they may only produce one dirty poop diaper per day. The parameters on what is normal and what is not are quite wide though so I have broken them down for you.

Frequency

In the first few days of your baby's life, they will probably poop once for every day of their life. This is especially true for breastfed babies and the pattern will be one poop for the first day of their life, two for the second, and so on until around the tenth day when things will even out and they will begin to poop less. Breastfed babies will have a change in their bowel patterns and consistency around six weeks old as your breastmilk changes to accommodate the next phase of their life and they may go a day or two without soiling their diaper with poop. Formula-fed babies can poop three or four times a day but can sometimes go just as long (three or four days) without soiling their diapers. If your baby has not pooped in more than four days, is lifting their legs, straining, or crying when pushing, they may be constipated and will need a pediatrician approved stool loosener to help their digestive system along.

What is Normal

The first few weeks of your baby's life will see a lot of changes in the color, consistency, and amount of poop they produce. The first poop they pass will be thick, tar-like, and be black, dark green, and sticky. This is called meconium, and your baby's first few poops may take on this color or consistency before changing to bright yellow, or yellow/brown, or mustard colored. Babies who breastfeed will normally tend to have more yellow or bright yellow bowel movements, where formula-fed babies will tend to have yellow to brown poop. Breastfed babies may also look like they have seeds in their poop and it may be more runny rather than paste-like. As your baby grows, their stool will change. Teething may cause bouts of runny poop which burns your baby's behind and, as you begin to introduce solids, you will see consistency, and smell changes. Some pieces of food may be present in newly introduced solids babies which is completely normal. Changes in your diet or your baby's diet will almost always change the color and consistency of their poop, and you will need to be aware of what you eat when breastfeeding and checking your little one's poop.

The normal color for your baby's poop can range from light yellow, bright yellow, dark green due to iron in formula, light brown, and medium to dark brown. Consistency can be runny and watery to a thick paste.

What is Not Normal

Red stool may not always be a problem, especially if you have recently introduced solids into your baby's diet which include beets or other foods in red color. Bright red or blood-stained poop needs to be seen by your pediatrician as it can be an indicator of intestinal bleeding.

Black poop is also not always a cause for alarm. Formula-fed babies and babies on iron supplements may have black or very dark green poop. This is due to the iron reacting internally with your baby's body. If your baby is not formula-fed, is not on iron supplements or their poop is pitch black, contact your pediatrician as this is a sign of upper digestive tract bleeding.

Bright green or olive green are not usually great signs of digestive health. If your baby's poop is green, watery, or runny, has mucus in the poop, they seem to be cramping and have had more diapers than normal there is probably a stomach bug brewing. Babies dehydrate incredibly quickly and even a suspected stomach bug should be treated by a healthcare professional.

Light-colored poop that has undigested formula in it should be reported to your doctor. It is normal for some undigested formula to pass through your baby's digestive tract if they are recovering from a stomach bug but the consistent presence of formula in your baby's poop could be a sign that your baby is not getting enough nutrition and there is a problem with their digestive tract.

White, or light grey stools should always be reported to your pediatrician or healthcare physician. Certain medications may cause white, clay-like poop but, more commonly, it is a sign that something is wrong with your baby's liver.

If you suspect there is an issue with your baby and you have picked it up through the color and consistency of their poop, be sure to take photos, or better yet, keep a fresh sample of their poop to take with you to the doctor's office.

Diapering

Changing your baby's diaper is not going to be one of your favorite parenting jobs but it is a necessity that will take up a whole lot of your time. Changing a diaper may seem like a simple enough task but did you know that there is a difference when cleaning your boy or girl baby's genital areas?

The basics are fairly easy, and if you have followed our what to have and getting ready sections of this book you should have all the tools available to change your baby's diaper quickly and efficiently. At every diaper change you will need a clean diaper, clean damp cotton wool, or a clean moist washcloth, or hypoallergenic newborn wipes, a change of clothing, in case your little one has pooped or wet through, a clean waterproof if you are using cloth diapers, diaper barrier cream or rash cream if your baby has a diaper rash. It will not take you long to figure out if your baby has pooped or peed their diaper as moms have an amazing built-in sense of smell which allows them to pick up their baby's scent, even in a large group of other baby's. Don't worry if you haven't already developed this; your baby will let you know that they need changing.

Begin by laying your baby on their back on their changing area, if they are high up use safety straps or have your hand on your baby at all times to prevent falls. Undo their current dirty diaper, wiping as much poop away as possible with the front inner part of the diaper. Diapers that have only been peed in can be folded underneath your baby. Poop skin will need to be thoroughly cleaned with wipes or a wet washcloth. Be sure to get into your little one's folds, lifting their legs to get underneath their behind. Once they are clean, you can slide the solid diaper out, place the new diaper under them, and apply whatever barrier cream or rash cream you are using before doing up their diaper and redressing your baby.

Diapering Your Baby Boy

While cleaning between the folds may be easier for little boys, they have an uncanny ability to pee as soon as their penis feels fresh air. As a mom of many boys, I can tell you that, without a doubt, you will be peed on at least once in your baby's early months and most times these fountains of pee come with hysterical giggles. To try and avoid being the target of your little boy's fountain, put a clean wipe or washcloth over their penis or watch for the beginnings of an erection to avoid disaster. Don't be afraid to clean around the penis and scrotum but do not pull on or try to retract your baby boy's foreskin. Pointing their penis downwards towards their scrotum will help prevent front spill disasters when your baby boys inevitably pees up their front.

86

Diapering Your Baby Girl

Your little girl will need special care when changing their diaper. Their little vagina has been wonderfully made to protect itself from poop entering the sensitive internal areas but you will need to ensure that poop diapers are changed quickly to avoid poop getting in the folds. When changing your little girl's diaper, ensure that you always wipe from front to back to avoid inadvertently transferring poop between their labia. You will not need to open your baby girl's labia to clean inside, even if you see some discharge. If they have had a particularly messy poop and you feel that you cannot safely change their diaper, you can always tail wash your little girl to get rid of any residue poop. Barrier cream and diaper rash cream should only be applied externally unless directed differently by your pediatrician. Never insert anything into your baby girl's vagina.

The Modern Diaper Movement

Being a mom in today's day and age has us spoiled for choice when it comes to diapers. Whether you decide to cloth diaper or disposable diaper is entirely up to you. Each diapering choice comes with pros and cons and when you make your choice you will need to weigh those pros and cons up.

Cloth Diapering

The average American family will spend between $750 and $1500 (US) per year on disposable diapers. This makes a very expensive exercise just to keep your little one's behind clean. In the past, cloth diapers needed to be folded before use and while that is still the case for some cloth diapers, most are easy to wash and prep for use. Most cloth diapers will come with a shell, inner, and locking system. While cloth diapers may cost more initially, over time you will recoup your investment and will save in the long run. Some cloth diapering systems are designed to expand with your little one and can be used from birth to potty training stage. To prevent staining, microfiber inserts can be used. Many of these cloth diaper options can be used as swim diapers as well. The disadvantage of cloth diapering is, of course, the need to wash dirty diapers constantly. This may become tedious and storing dirty diapers that need to be washed when out and about can be a bit of a challenge. Should you decide to go with a cloth diapering solution, ensure that you have sufficient inners, waterproofs, and liners to cover rainy day missed washes and times where your little one may have more poops than usual.

Disposable Diapering

As we mentioned before, disposable diapering is expensive but is convenient. Modern disposable diapers usually come with wetness indicator strips which allow moms to know exactly how much liquid your baby's diaper is holding. Aside from the obvious convenience of having a diaper that does not need to be washed, most disposable diapers come with built-in dermatological protection for your little one's soft behind. The disadvantage to disposable diapers is that they aren't great for the environment and when you do the maths, diapering one baby can mean contributing to an already bad environmental situation.

Chapter 7: Common Issues

Even the easiest babies can give their mom a little bit of trouble from time to time. Whether this is with feeding, spit-up issues, or sleep regression, the occasional hiccup along the way can be overcome.

Breastfeeding

Of the issues moms face most, breastfeeding is probably top of the list. Breastfeeding requires a massive commitment from the mom and can come with a set of issues that may seem overwhelmingly difficult to fix. The good news is that, with a little persistence and sometimes a tweak or change here and there, these issues can be fixed, setting you back on the path of easier feeding.

Sore Nipples

Most women will tell you that sore nipples are the reason they quit breastfeeding. While it is true that there will be times where breastfeeding will feel uncomfortable, feeding should not be painful. Sometimes, all it takes is a little time for your nipples to toughen but, most of the time, pain during breastfeeding means that your baby's latch is incorrect and they are injuring you. To correct this, you can try and separate your baby from your breast by placing your clean baby finger into the corner of their mouth, unlatching and then relatching them to your breast. If your breasts are still painful and your baby persistently latches incorrectly, speak to your local lactation specialist to help your baby to latch correctly.

Breast Engorgement

Your breasts will engorge as your milk comes in, around three days after birth. Your breasts may feel hard, extremely sore and you may sweat profusely and leak milk. The good news is that this phase only lasts about two days before it corrects itself. In the meantime, try to put your little one on the breast as often as possible, stand next to them when they cry to encourage the letdown response, use a warm to hot cloth to encourage let-down, and apply cold cabbage leaves or compresses to your breasts to relieve the pain. While breast engorgement is uncomfortable, it is a necessary part of breastfeeding and, with a suckling baby and the help of hand expression, it will pass quickly.

Leaking

Your breasts need time to adjust to the supply and demand of your baby and, because of that, you can pretty much spring a leak at any time and any place. Make sure that you have an adequate supply of breast pads, pump often to prevent leaks, and double up on protection until your breasts have become accustomed to breastfeeding.

Milk Ducts that are Clogged or Infected

Milk ducts can become clogged as a result of milk that has backed up. While clogged milk ducts are not serious, it can be uncomfortable and may lead to an infection if it is not treated. Try to apply a warm cloth to the duct, massage it often and breastfeed as often as possible. Most times, the duct will unclog itself but if you suspect an infection or the lump will not drain or move after three days, consult your physician or lactation specialist.

Mastitis

Also referred to as milk fever, mastitis is serious and needs to be corrected promptly by your physician. Trapped milk can lead to an infection in your breast or breasts. This causes a high fever, flu-like symptoms, red inflamed breasts, muscle pain, and breast pain. Your doctor will need to prescribe baby-friendly antibiotics and a pain reliever to help you overcome the infection and relieve the pain you are in.

Tongue-Tie and Other Palate Issues

Sometimes your baby may be born with a mouth deformity that cannot be seen. Many times your lactation specialist or the nurse in the hospital will pick up there is a problem long before you do. If your baby is clicking their tongue when latching, gulping exorbitant amounts of air, seems to not be able to latch at all, or is making kissing sounds when drinking, chances are they have a congenital deformity of the mouth or tongue. While this sounds scary, oftentimes it will not cause issues later in life. Some of these issues can be corrected with latch position changing and others will mean that your baby will need to use specialist bottles to help them to latch properly. It may be frustrating for you that your baby cannot feed directly from the breast but it doesn't make you any less of a great mom, and as long as your baby is being fed, you are doing the best you can for them.

Spit-Up

About 50% of baby's spit-up with breastfed babies spitting up less than bottle-fed babies. This happens when your baby gulps air down when feeding. When your baby's stomach is full or you change their position abruptly after feeding, they will spit up some of their milk because the tiny valve that stops food from entering the esophagus is not yet properly developed. Some babies will spit-up more than others and the amount of spit-up can look scary but if your baby is not violently throwing up, displaying discomfort, or is not picking up weight, chances are that they are spitting up a normal amount. A baby who spits up a little bit or mostly feeds probably has a little bit of gastroesophageal reflux and there is nothing much you can do. If your baby is a quick guzzler, sucks in a lot of air, or tends to be hyper-excited, you can try some of the tips and tricks given in the 'feeding' section of this book.

There are some issues to look out for though when feeding your baby. Spit-up which is accompanied by muscle spasms or contraction, that comes out with force, or a large amount of spit-up that seems to be the majority or all of your baby's feed is an indicator of a much larger problem. As mentioned before, babies dehydrate incredibly quickly and a loss of fluid through vomiting requires a visit to your pediatrician or emergency room. Signs of dehydration include fewer wet diapers or no wet diaper within a two hour period, crying without tears, skin which does not go back to its position when lightly pinched, and a sunken soft spot. If your baby shows any of these signs, do not wait. Take them to the emergency room for immediate attention. Blood in your baby's spit-up could be an indication of a bigger problem as well and will require a diagnosis from your doctor.

While spitting-up is normal for most babies, there are some tips and tricks to help reduce the amount of spit-up your baby produces. Avoid overfeeding, or tank feeding your baby, slow their feeds by interrupting their feed to wind them, feed your baby smaller amounts, more frequently and try to feed them in a slightly more upright position but never sitting up. If your baby is still spitting-up a large amount after trying all of these tricks, consider changing something in your diet, if you are breastfeeding, or consider changing your baby's formula. True reflux or GERD is very rare in babies and your pediatrician will be able to guide you in the right direction when it comes to anti-reflux formulas or breast milk thickening agents. Do not add cereal or oatmeal to your baby's bottle as this can cause choking.

Sleep Issues

Sleeping and the issues surrounding it have been covered in the 'sleeping' section of this book but did you know there could be other reasons why your baby is not sleeping?

Your baby may be suffering from separation anxiety! From as early as four months old, your baby may realize that you are not around when they drift off to sleep and this may leave them feeling anxious and fighting off sleep. Separation anxiety usually peaks between the ages of six and nine months in babies and can lead to your little one waking often, over-stimulating themselves, or even crying themselves to sleep. If your baby is crying for none of the reasons we have already listed, does not have a medical problem, and has had colic ruled out of the equation, chances are that they are crying just to summon you. Easing your baby out of separation anxiety can be tough on both mom and baby but with a little persistence, it can be beaten. The important thing is to remain calm, soothing your baby with your voice and touch, reassuring them that you are still present, even when they are asleep. You will need to be consistent in your soothing behavior as babies learn from repetitive actions, especially after the age of six months. Rest assured that, with some consistency, a little patience, and a whole lot of your loving touch, your baby will transition into this phase relatively quickly.

Chapter 8: Common Illnesses

Being outside of the womb means that your little one is being exposed to new viruses, bacteria, and germs daily. Because of this, they are bound to get sick at some point and you will need to be prepared. While good hygiene prevents a host of germs from entering your baby's body all at once, some exposure to the outside world will be needed to build up their immune system and help them to fight off sickness later in life.

Vaccination

Aside from breastfeeding, to vaccinate or not to vaccinate is the most hotly debated topic amongst moms. If your baby was born in a hospital, chances are they have already received their first vaccinations, unless you specifically requested that they do not receive them. You will need to educate yourself and gain all of the facts regarding vaccination to make the right decision for you and your baby.

Vaccines are designed to prevent or ease the symptoms of common dangerous and sometimes deadly diseases. All of the ingredients in your baby's vaccinations should be made available to you upon request which will allow you to put your mind at rest that vaccination is the right choice for you. Vaccines work by building your baby's immune system allowing it to fend off diseases when they are exposed to them. And, whether you like it or not, your baby will be exposed to germs no matter how fastidious you are about health and hygiene in your home. When you vaccinate your baby, a minuscule amount of antigen, the germ you are vaccinating against, enters your baby's bloodstream triggering their immune response, and helping the body to recognize the germ the next time your baby is exposed to it. In the same way that you buckle your baby in every time you go for a drive without expecting to have an accident, vaccination protects your baby in the event that he or she is exposed to the disease While there may be horror stories all over the internet about the side effects of vaccines, the reality is that severe side effects are few and far between. To put your mind at rest when researching vaccination, always ensure that you are looking up information on credible websites that verify their information with facts and figures. Your baby may suffer some minor side effects, including a low fever, some localized injection site pain, a slight rash, and redness around the site of the vaccination. These can all be managed at home with the use of pediatrician recommended pain and fever medications. On the off chance that your baby does have a severe reaction to their vaccination, take them to the emergency room immediately and advise the attending healthcare professional of the vaccine and any medications you have given your baby.

Common Baby Ailments

Many common baby illnesses and ailments can be managed at home with a little tender loving care, approved pediatric over-the-counter medication, and the right amount of feeding and rest. Some of these common baby ailments include:

Low-Grade Fever

A fever is the body's natural response to fighting off an infection or a germ that has entered the system with the intent to make a person sick. Everyone will at some point in their life develop a fever, and often with baby's that fever will develop at night when your baby is resting. Because of this, you should always have and know the location of your thermometer and pediatric medication.

A normal human body temperature is 98.6 degrees Fahrenheit or 36.8 degrees centigrade. Naturally, a person's temperature may fluctuate by a few points but a dip or rise of more than 0.5 degrees could be an indication that an infection is brewing. Because your baby has not yet learned how to regulate their body temperature, over or underdressing them may cause rapid fluctuations in their body temperature and you should first ensure that your baby is not too hot or too cold before assuming they are sick. Teething may cause your baby's temperature to rise but this should not be a significant temperature rise and anything more than one degree higher than normal in an infant under the age of six months is considered a medical emergency.

Signs of a fever include a temperature of more than 100.4 degrees Fahrenheit or 38 degrees centigrade, cold and clammy skin or skin that feels hot to the touch, red, bloodshot eyes, general fussiness, dehydration, and drowsiness. Low-grade fevers of under 102 degrees Fahrenheit can be treated at home by keeping your baby cool, administering pediatric fever medication every four to six hours, and offering more frequent small feeds to keep hydration levels up. Infants under the age of three months with a temperature of more than 100.4 degrees should be seen by a doctor immediately, and anything over this is considered a medical emergency. If your baby has had a fever for more than 24 hours, or if they seem excessively lethargic, or if you have trouble waking them, make an appointment to see your healthcare physician immediately.

Eye Discharge and Drainage

It is fairly common for babies to have discharge and some drainage issues relating to the tear ducts in the first few weeks of their lives. As the tear ducts develop, and as they become accustomed to external eye irritants, these drainage issues will disappear and, if they do not, your pediatrician will recommend a minor procedure to open the tear ducts. To encourage movement through the tear duct, gentle pressure can be placed on the side of the nose, moving your finger in an upward and outward direction towards the tear duct. Do not place too much pressure on your baby's nose or face and do not touch your baby's eye. Should any white or milky discharge move out of the tear duct, you can gently wipe it away with a warm, wet cotton pad.

Discharge that becomes yellow or green, eyelids that are stuck together after sleeping, and continual discharge may be a sign of bacterial or viral infection of the eyes or the tear ducts. Should your baby have signs of an infection or have persistently blocked tear ducts, you will need to contact your healthcare physician for an appointment to ensure that the infection does not spread to the sinus area.

The Common Cold

We've all had one at least once in our lives, and as your baby's immune system still needs to develop, they can be susceptible to viral infections that cause the common cold. While a cold is not serious, it can make your baby fussy and miserable and, if not treated properly, may develop into more serious bacterial infections.

Symptoms of a cold in your baby will start with fussiness and a running nose and may progress to a low-grade fever, coughing which escalates at night, issues falling asleep or frequent wakings, difficulty feeding, or not wanting to feed. Common colds should be treated at home with the help of pediatric inhalants to relieve your baby's cough, and fever and pain medication to help ease the discomfort associated with a cold, as well as nasal suctioning, or saline solution to keep your baby's nose clear of excess mucus.

You will need to keep an eye on your baby to ensure that the infection does not progress. If your baby develops a high fever, has mucus that turns yellow or green, is showing signs of respiratory distress, has a cough that makes it difficult for them to breathe, or you have trouble waking them and they are unresponsive, you will need to see your pediatrician immediately. Babies under the age of three months should be seen by your healthcare physician to ensure that no infection is brewing. For babies over three months old, signs of infection or a fever of 101 degrees Fahrenheit warrant a visit to your doctor. A cold which lasts more than five days is a sign of a more serious infection and needs to be seen by a physician. Never give your baby cold and flu medication without the express direction of your physician.

Vomiting and Diarrhea

A little spit-up and runny poop is all part and parcel of being a baby. Between three and six months your baby might go through periods where their poop seems more liquid, or they may seem to spit-up more often. This is all completely normal as their digestive system gets used to different feeding patterns, milk changes, growth spurts, and those dreaded teeth. If your baby's stomach is violently contracting, spit-up comes out with force, and they are crying because of muscle spasms they are no longer spitting up but are vomiting.

Likewise, running poop with a little bit of slime in it is not something to be concerned about unless your baby has had more than two running, slimy poops, seems to be having stomach cramps, or their poop has turned green suddenly and contains lumps of undigested milk or formula.

Vomiting and diarrhea can come with or without a fever and maybe be a sign of viral or bacterial infection, trouble digesting new food or food allergies. Persistent vomiting and diarrhea are classified as more than two consecutive diarrhea diapers and two violent vomiting episodes in which the content of your baby's stomach is emptied. True vomiting and diarrhea are extremely dangerous in babies. This is especially true for babies under the age of three months, and should be treated as a medical emergency. While waiting to see a doctor, or while on your way to the emergency room, try and offer your baby more feeds than normal, even if they are sipping on milk, they are getting some nourishment and hydration. Never withhold food or milk from your vomiting baby.

Ear Infections

Classified as an inflammation of the middle ear, ear infections can be the result of a variety of causes. Generally, infections present themselves when fluid backs up behind the eardrum and bacteria begin to breed. Ear infections are incredibly common, and five in six children will have at least one ear infection before their toddler years.

In babies, ear infections are difficult to identify as it may seem your little one is teething or is generally unwell. There are, however, some telltale signs that your baby has an ear infection. These include a flushed cheek on the infected ear side, pulling or putting their fingers in their ears, crying when laid down flat, fussiness and crying when feeding, an inability to settle when they sleep, good or fluid coming from the ear, and sometimes a fever.

Ear infections are incredibly uncomfortable for your baby, and if you have ruled out teething as the cause of your baby's discomfort, you should make an appointment to see your doctor. The American Paediatric Academy recommends that all babies under the age of six months should be seen by a physician if the parents suspect their child has an ear infection because ear infections can spike a baby's fever very quickly, and may cause permanent damage to your baby's hearing if fluid and bacteria are left to back up behind the eardrum. In the meantime, try and keep your baby elevated at a 45-degree angle when sleeping to prevent discomfort but keep an eye on their breathing and ensure that their head does not flop or lull forward. Do not expose your baby to second-hand smoke, or feed them laying completely prone as these are the leading causes of ear infections in babies.

Falls and Lacerations

Fall safety should be practiced at all times with your baby, diaper changes, and bathing should be done with safety straps or with your hand on your baby at all times, but accidents do happen. The most common cause of head bumps and lacerations in infants comes when they are a little older and begin to explore the world with their mouths. Add teeth to the equation and your little one may end up bumping their mouths or head on any number of objects as they learn the limitations of what the outside world has to offer. Added to this, your baby's head makes up most of their body weight and a topple will almost always result in them landing headfirst.

The most common fall hazards for your little one are stairs, your bed or theirs, windows, baths, changing tables, and baby walkers. Little ones learn in leaps and bounds! Yesterday, they couldn't roll and today they are rolling like a pro. If an accident does happen, you must remain calm. Your baby will scream, and will in all likeliness lose their breath as a result of the knock, pain, and shock. Assess the situation. Has your baby landed on their head? Are they acting strangely? Are they bleeding? Have they gone underwater in the tub? Babies who are under three months should be seen by a doctor immediately if they have hit their head or their neck has bent backward or forwards violently. If your baby is over three months you will need to calmly assess the injury. Knocks on your baby's mouth and minor knocks on the front or back of their head are going to be part of the learning process as they begin to sit, roll, and mouth their way through life. Trust your instincts! If you think something is wrong or your baby is acting strangely after a fall, you're probably right and should visit the emergency room.

Deep lacerations and cuts should be treated with firm pressure to stem bleeding, and you should contact your emergency room or department immediately. Light cuts and bruises can be treated at home with warm and cold compresses and a little pediatric ointment to prevent infection.

All burns should be seen by a physician as burned skin allows bacteria to easily enter your baby's system and may result in secondary infections. To treat burns while you wait for your doctor, apply some breast milk to the site, or use a room temperature compress to soothe the burn. If your baby has been burned badly and the skin is open, or blistering, do not apply anything to the wound. Call emergency services immediately so that they can use correct burn treatment wound care equipment.

If your baby falls from a height, knocks their head violently, has fallen into water, or is vomiting and acting disoriented after a fall, seek immediate medical care!

Remember that accidents happen, mom, and most of the time it will not be your fault.

Chapter 9: Top Questions From New Moms

Being a mom means constantly asking questions. Babies are all so unique that even the most seasoned moms will be stumped from time to time and will need to seek the guidance of others to navigate parenthood. As a new mom, you will have a whole lot of questions, from how often to feed your baby to if you will ever sleep again.

Birth

Q. Does birth hurt?

In a word? Yes. Whether you opt for a natural unmedicated birth, cesarean or epidural, birth comes with some level of pain and discomfort during your recovery period. The good news is that this pain is temporary, and with the help of approved pain medications, is manageable.

Q. Will I poop on the table?

Maybe. It is quite common for first time, and even seasoned moms to confuse the perineal muscles with the muscles that help you to pass a bowel movement. Some moms will be given a laxative in the beginning stages of labor to clean their system out, some may develop diarrhea a day or two before birth, and some may poop on the table. Rest assured that doctors and midwives have seen it all, and you probably won't even be aware of the fact that you have had a bowel movement. No one will tell you in any case so don't worry about it.

Q. Am I less of a woman for having a cesarean?

Absolutely not! Birth is birth, momma, and you will have your own memorable experience regardless of whether or not you decide on natural birth.

Q. Is birth really that much of a privacy invasion?

Yes! And you won't care. Regardless of whether you have a natural birth or not, your entire lower end will be exposed and there will be numerous people present. Your nerves and excitement at meeting your baby will mean you just don't care. Your modesty can return much later.

Q. Will my baby be placed on my chest at birth?

Maybe. This is very much dependent on the type of birth you have and whether there are any complications. For the most part, an uncomplicated natural birth will mean that your baby can be placed directly on your chest straight after birth. If you choose to have a cesarean, or if there are complications at birth, chances are you will be shown your baby briefly before your healthcare professionals attend to sewing you up, or to your baby's needs.

Postpartum

Q. How long will I bleed?

Postpartum bleeding is referred to as lochlea and can last anywhere from four to 12 weeks. If you give birth in a hospital, you will be closely monitored for large clots and excessive bleeding.

Q. When should I be concerned about my bleeding?

By Day 10, your bleeding should have tapered off from heavy to medium-light flow. If your bleeding increases, if you pass clots bigger than the size of a grape, if your bleeding smells bad, or if your bleeding changes color from pink, yellow, or brown back to bright red contact your health care physician or midwife immediately. Postpartum hemorrhage is a rare but serious postpartum complication that needs to be attended to immediately.

Q. Will I ever look the same again?

Chances are no. Your body will change, some of those changes will be good, and some of them you may not like. Maintaining a healthy diet, taking time to heal, and embracing your new body will go a long way in helping you to embrace the new you.

Q. How long will I take to recover?

There is no definitive answer to that question. Some moms bounce back quickly, some take a little longer. Remember that you grew an entire human being for nine months and you birthed them. Be patient with yourself, it may take some time but you will find your mojo again.

Q. Will I ever get my life back?

This is a double-edged sword. The true answer is no, but your new life will be different, sometimes chaotic, and almost certainly filled with the most gorgeous gummy smiles and new quirks as your baby grows and develops their personality. Finding a routine that works well for you and your baby, and sticking to it will help you adjust to your new normal life.

Q. Will my vagina be different?

No. Initially you will be swollen, tender, may have stitches or slight lacerations, and will need some time to have things return back to the way they were before. As your body heals, and as your hormones begin to stabilize once more, your vagina will return to the way it was before. Remember that your body is designed to birth a baby and your vagina has the amazing ability to stretch and return to its normal size and shape.

Q. When will I get my sex drive back?

You have given birth to a baby and will spend at least the next six weeks elbow deep in poop, spit-up, and nighttime feeds. Be patient with yourself through the exhaustion, and the flurry of hormones. Some women are ready for sex as early as six weeks, others take a full year to recover. Be open and honest with your partner about your feelings on sex and be patient with yourself. You will not be celibate forever.

Q. When will I get my first period?

You are fertile as early as two weeks after birth and this means that your first period may come back as soon as four to six weeks after giving birth to your baby. Breastfeeding moms generally take longer to have their menstrual cycle return normally but may still be fertile no matter how much your grandmother insists that breastfeeding as a contraceptive. If you do not want to fall pregnant straight away, speak to your healthcare professional about breastfeeding safe contraceptive options.

Newborn

Q. Should I swaddle my newborn?

Maybe. It is entirely up to you and your baby if swaddling works. Some babies love the feeling of being swaddled, while others may hate it. If you do decide to swaddle your baby, always put them down to sleep on their back and do not swaddle over the age of three months.

Q. Can I leave my newborn to sleep through the night?

No. Your baby will need to be woken every two to three hours to be fed.

Q. Why is my newborn squinting?

A baby's vision is not yet fully developed and because of that, they will squint to try and focus and because they do not yet have full control over the optic muscles. If your baby's eyes return to their normal position relatively quickly, this is completely normal.

Feeding, Spit-up, and Poop

Q. Should I wake my sleeping baby to feed them?

Yes. At least for the first three months of your baby's life, they should be woken every two to three hours for a feed. After three months, nighttime feeds may be stretched to between four and five hours and by six months you can allow your baby to go a full eight hours at night as long as they are feeding frequently during the day.

Q. How long should I breastfeed my baby?

This is entirely up to you. Some moms feed for the first few days of their newborn's life while others feed well into the toddler years. If you have a condition, are on medication, or suffer from a disease that prevents breastfeeding, speak to your healthcare provider for information and advice on which formula will work best for your baby.

Q. How often does my baby need to be fed?

Initially, your baby will need to be fed every two to three hours, but the time period will begin to stretch as your baby gets older. Consult the comprehensive feeding chapter of this book for more information.

Q. Should I worry that my baby is spitting up?

No. A little bit of spit-up is completely normal. For more information on your baby and spit-up, consult the comprehensive spit-up chapter of this book.

Q. Why is my baby's poop a weird color?

Baby poop comes in all manner of color, odor, and texture. Consult our 'scoop on poop', section for more information.

Q. How often will my baby poop?

Often, to begin with. Initially, your baby will poop for every day of their lives until they are 12 days old. That means one poop for day one, two for day two, and so on until they reach approximately two weeks old. Consult our 'scoop on poop' chapter of this book for more information.

Illnesses

Q. When should I call the doctor?

If your baby has fallen and hit their head, if they have a fever, if they are showing signs of respiratory distress, or if your instincts are telling you something isn't right with your baby, don't hesitate to contact your doctor.

Q. What should I do if my baby has a fever?

A fever of over 100.4 degrees Fahrenheit or 38 degrees centigrade is a medical emergency and requires immediate medical attention. Consult the chapter on common illnesses for more information.

Q. My baby is only six weeks old, why does it look like they are teething?

Babies can begin teething as early as six weeks old. If your baby is showing signs of teething, is drooling excessively, and is generally fussy, chances are you have an early teether.

Conclusion

Becoming a mom is such an amazing event in your life. It is one that will change you and your life forever and, while it may seem tough and overwhelming to begin with, will bring you some of the most joyful moments of your life. Diving into the internet for information can be helpful but with so many articles out there, all expressing their own opinion, being lost in the web of information may have you feeling like you just aren't ready for this at all.

While it is true that the first few months of parenthood are not for the faint-hearted, some things can make the transition easier. Honestly, being a mom means relying on your instincts and your gut far more than that 'rock and slide', or any perfect plan you may have for you and your baby. Every baby is different, and no list will ever give you a comprehensive idea of what mommyhood will look like to you. You will spend a whole lot of time preparing for your baby's arrival, and some of those preparations may come to fruition while some may fall to pieces as your tiny tyke demands for you to know that they are an individual. Broken plans or contrary routines combined with hormones and exhaustion can feel soul-crushing but take the lead from your baby and gently guide them into a routine that works for you both. Create a birth plan, then create an opposite birth plan. Create a feeding schedule and then create the exact opposite of that schedule. The same goes for sleeping schedules, bathing schedules, and going out because the wheels will fall off the bus at some point, and being prepared for the unexpected is what is going to get you through the first few months with your little one.

Understand that bonding may take a little bit of time and that is okay! Not every mom will have that awe-inspiring feeling of an instant connection with their baby but with a little bit of time, patience, and understanding, that bond will come. Talking about time, you're going to have very little of it to begin with and, because of that, you should reach out to your friends and family for as much or as little help as you need. If someone offers to bring over dinner or to watch the baby for a few minutes while you shower, say yes. You will be grateful for it later. I promise. Having a good support structure of over-enthusiastic helpers and people you can call on when you feel like a weepy mess will be the single most valuable resource available to you as you navigate the first few weeks of being a mom. Never feel ashamed of asking for help, it takes a village, and sometimes, a little medication and therapy to raise a baby. You will need to give yourself six months to a year to truly get into the swing of things, not just your body but adjusting to your new normal life.

Understand that breastfeeding is hard and while it is recommended, it is not for everyone. Formula feeding your baby does not make you any less of a mom. A happy mom is a happy baby and as long as your little one is fed well, there is absolutely nothing wrong with the choice you have made. Comparing yourself to other moms is not fair to you. You are as unique as your baby and, as the saying goes, 'all roads lead to Rome'.

Invest the time and money you would have spent on items that are needed, on making your environment comfortable to allow for bonding together. The single most valuable item I purchased as a mom was my baby wrap; it allowed me to wear my baby while I got my life back, knowing he was safe, secure, and felt loved being so close to me. Find what works for you when trying to find your feet and stick to it. It may seem overwhelming now but this too shall pass momma, and before you know it, your whole new life will have begun.

References

7 of the most common childhood injuries and accidents (and when specialized emergency care may be needed). (2020, July 28). HealthPartners Blog. https://www.healthpartners.com/blog/most-common-childhood-injuries/

20 common questions from new parents, answered by a pediatrician. (2018, July 4). Moms. https://www.moms.com/20-common-questions-from-new-parents-answered-by-a-pediatrician/

23 popular baby items you should stay away from -. (2020, August 20). https://wholesomechildren.com/baby-items-you-dont-need/

Advice for new mothers on getting to know your newborn baby. Breastfeeding Tips and Breast Pump Info for Moms from Medela Canada. http://www.medelabreastfeedingtips.ca/advice-for-new-mothers-on-getting-to-know-your-newborn-baby/

_ApplicationFrame. (n.d.). Children's Minnesota. https://www.childrensmn.org/educationmaterials/childrensmn/article/15276/infant-behavior-cues/

Baby. (n.d.). HealthyChildren.org. Retrieved January 16, 2021, from https://healthychildren.org/English/ages-stages/baby/Pages/default.aspx

Bathing your baby. (n.d.). HealthyChildren.org. https://www.healthychildren.org/English/ages-stages/baby/bathing-skin-care/Pages/Bathing-Your-Newborn.aspx

Bowel movements in babies. (n.d.). HealthLink BC. Retrieved January 16, 2021, from https://www.healthlinkbc.ca/health-topics/abo3062

CDC. (2019, August 5). *Making the vaccine decision: Common concerns.* Centers for Disease Control and Prevention. https://www.cdc.gov/vaccines/parents/why-vaccinate/vaccine-decision.html

Dewar, G. (2019). *Infant sleep problems: A troubleshooting guide.* Parentingscience.com; Parenting Science. https://www.parentingscience.com/infant-sleep-problems.html

Ear infections in children. (2015, August 18). NIDCD. https://www.nidcd.nih.gov/health/ear-infections-children

Eye—pus or discharge. (n.d.). Seattle Children's Hospital. https://www.seattlechildrens.org/conditions/a-z/eye-pus-or-discharge/

Feeding patterns: My nursing coach. (n.d.). Www.Mynursingcoach.com. Retrieved January 16, 2021, from https://www.mynursingcoach.com/feeding-patterns/

Feeding your newborn (for parents)—Nemours KidsHealth. (n.d.). Kidshealth.org. https://kidshealth.org/en/parents/feednewborn.html

Fevers. (2018). Kidshealth.org. https://kidshealth.org/en/parents/fever.html

Getting to know your newborn. (2020, December 8). Nhs.Uk. https://www.nhs.uk/pregnancy/labour-and-birth/after-the-birth/getting-to-know-your-newborn/

Health, D. (2011). *The importance of infant bonding | UC Davis Medical Center.* Ucdavis.Edu.

https://health.ucdavis.edu/medicalcenter/healthtips/20100114_infant-bonding.html

Home. (2019). Zero to three. https://www.zerotothree.org/

Homepage | La Leche League International. (2017). La Leche League International. https://www.llli.org/

How can you get your baby on a feeding schedule? (n.d.). Healthline. https://www.healthline.com/health/parenting/baby-feeding-schedule

Medicine cabinet checklist. (n.d.). WebMD. Retrieved January 16, 2021, from https://www.webmd.com/baby/medicine-cabinet-checklist

Modern cloth diapering {all you need to know} ~ A complete guide. (2014, April 21). Jornie. https://jornie.com/cloth-diapering/

Newborn archives • KellyMom.com. (n.d.). KellyMom.com. Retrieved January 16, 2021, from https://kellymom.com/category/ages/newborn

Newborn sleep patterns. (n.d.). Www.Hopkinsmedicine.org. https://www.hopkinsmedicine.org/health/wellness-and-prevention/newborn-sleep-patterns

POSTPARTUM PROGRESS | postpartum depression and postpartum anxiety help for moms. (n.d.). POSTPARTUM PROGRESS. Retrieved January 16, 2021, from https://postpartumprogress.com/

Sleep 0—3 months. (n.d.). Healthywa.Wa.Gov.Au. https://healthywa.wa.gov.au/Articles/S_T/Sleep-0-3-months

Sleep and your newborn (for parents)—Nemours KidsHealth. (n.d.). Kidshealth.org. https://kidshealth.org/en/parents/sleepnewborn.html

Taylor, K. K. (2019, May 7). *Newborn essentials checklist: Save money with baby basics.* Squawkfox. https://www.squawkfox.com/newborn-essentials-checklist/

The 5 S's for baby: A guide for soothing your little one. (2020, June 18). Healthline. https://www.healthline.com/health/baby/5-s-baby

Today's Parent. (2020, January 7). *Newborn checklist: Everything you need before your baby arrives.* Today's Parent. https://www.todaysparent.com/checklists/newborn-checklist/

Umbilical care. (n.d.). Raising Children Network. https://raisingchildren.net.au/newborns/health-daily-care/hygiene-keeping-clean/umbilical-care

Why babies spit up. (n.d.). HealthyChildren.org. https://www.healthychildren.org/English/ages-stages/baby/feeding-nutrition/Pages/Why-Babies-Spit-Up.aspx

Made in the USA
Columbia, SC
30 July 2021